CURE CONSTIPATI

CURE
CONSTIPATION
NOW

A DOCTOR'S FIBER THERAPY TO CLEANSE AND HEAL

WITHDRAWN

Wes Jones,

M.D., FACP, AGAF

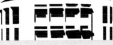

BERKLEY BOOKS, NEW YORK

THE BERKLEY PUBLISHING GROUP
Published by the Penguin Group
Penguin Group (USA) Inc.
375 Hudson Street, New York, New York 10014, USA
Penguin Group (Canada), 90 Eglinton Avenue East, Suite 700, Toronto, Ontario M4P 2Y3, Canada
(a division of Pearson Penguin Canada Inc.)
Penguin Books Ltd., 80 Strand, London WC2R 0RL, England
Penguin Group Ireland, 25 St. Stephen's Green, Dublin 2, Ireland (a division of Penguin Books Ltd.)
Penguin Group (Australia), 250 Camberwell Road, Camberwell, Victoria 3124, Australia
(a division of Pearson Australia Group Pty. Ltd.)
Penguin Books India Pvt. Ltd., 11 Community Centre, Panchsheel Park, New Delhi—110 017, India
Penguin Group (NZ), 67 Apollo Drive, Rosedale, North Shore 0632, New Zealand
(a division of Pearson New Zealand Ltd.)
Penguin Books (South Africa) (Pty.) Ltd., 24 Sturdee Avenue, Rosebank, Johannesburg 2196,
South Africa

Penguin Books Ltd., Registered Offices: 80 Strand, London WC2R 0RL, England

This book is an original publication of The Berkley Publishing Group.

Copyright © 2009 by Wes Jones, M.D.
Cover design by Lesley Worrell.
Interior text design by Richard Oriolo.

PRINTING HISTORY
Berkley trade paperback edition / July 2009

Library of Congress Cataloging-in-Publication Data

Jones, Wes, 1949–
    Cure constipation now : a doctor's fiber therapy to cleanse and heal / Wes Jones.
        p. cm.
    Includes bibliographical references and index.
    ISBN 978-0-425-22755-8
    1. Constipation.   2. High-fiber diet.   3. Colon (Anatomy)—Diseases.   I. Title.

    RC861.J668 2009
    616.3'428—dc22
    2009008915

PRINTED IN THE UNITED STATES OF AMERICA

10   9   8   7   6   5   4   3

PUBLISHER'S NOTE: Neither the publisher nor the author is engaged in rendering professional advice
or services to the individual reader. The ideas, procedures, and suggestions contained in this book are
not intended as a substitute for consulting with your physician. All matters regarding your health require
medical supervision. Neither the author nor the publisher shall be liable or responsible for any loss or
damage allegedly arising from any information or suggestion in this book.

The events described in this book are the real experiences of real people. However, the author has
altered their identities and, in some instances, created composite characters. Any resemblance between
a character in this book and a real person, therefore, is entirely accidental.

The publisher does not have any control over and does not assume any responsibility for author or third-
party websites or their content.

Contents

Acknowledgments

I am forever indebted to my patients for their forbearance in teaching me what worked and what did not work. Indeed, the fiber program that is the heart and soul of this book has been developed through a trial-and-error process, with my patients giving me the necessary feedback.

Equally important in making this book a reality has been my immediate family, especially Lucy, my wife, who has persevered throughout the long and arduous process of getting this book published. While I was busy with the book, Lucy focused her energies on finding an agent, writing the query letter, helping with the book proposal, and so forth. I must also express my sincere gratitude to Hollis, my eldest son and now a dentist, who helped me with earlier versions of this manuscript. While Hollis was involved with the creative side of the book, Jordan, my other son, was the "techie" who helped with most of the technical aspects of using the computer software, including procuring and setting up two laptops. Finally, "Rosie" (Rosanne), my daughter, allowed "her problem" (IBS) to be discussed in a public venue, so that teenagers might realize that help is available, if they would only look for answers. As Rosie said, "I kept thinking I could just deal with the problem. But I was wrong." This book clearly has been a team effort by our family.

I must also express my heartfelt gratitude to my partners at

Cape Fear Center for Digestive Diseases: Dr. Christian Chung, Dr. Rakesh Gupta, Dr. Sanjeev Slehria, Dr. Bryan Uslick, as well as Mrs. Kristin Russell, P.A., all of whom have supported me over the long years as the fiber program was developed and this book was written. I must especially thank my office nurses (past and present), but specifically Mrs. Tammy Godwin and Mrs. Nora Rachels, who have tirelessly reinforced the fiber message to my patients. Honorable mention also includes all the GI nurses with whom I work at various medical facilities, including my office, Highsmith-Rainey Specialty Hospital, Cape Fear Valley Health System, and the Fayetteville VA Hospital. Clearly, I could not get my message across to my patients without their support.

Dr. Stephen Logue requires my well-deserved gratitude for his enduring friendship, the fodder of material he provided for the book, and also his early recognition of the value of the fiber program for his patients. Equally important has been Dr. Henry Lesesne, gastroenterologist and professor of medicine at the University of North Carolina at Chapel Hill, who introduced me to the late Dr. Denis Burkitt's research, reinforcing my impression that the fiber story deserved a public forum. Also, I must thank Dr. Martin Poleski, gastroenterologist and professor of medicine at DUHS, who reviewed an earlier version of the book and provided encouragement. My sincere thanks also must be given to Dr. Esperanza Aid, Dr. Dardo Chávez Soleto, Dr. Martin Chipman, Dr. Henrique Echegaray Forest, Dr. Malcolm Fleishman, Dr. John Gimesh, Dr. Joel Horowitz, Dr. Victor Hugo Vásquez Lapaca, Dr. Weldon Jordan, and Dr. Paul Nordness, all of whom have either provided information, resources, or case histories for this book.

Ms. Jodie Rhodes, my agent, should be highlighted for her keen insight into the value of this book for the general public, for her ability to link me with Penguin, for her sage advice guiding me through the process of book publication, and finally for connecting me with Mrs. Deborah (Deb) Baker. I am equally indebted to Deb, my freelance editor, for her wise counsel and attention to detail and whose assistance greatly facilitated Penguin's acceptance of the manuscript for publication. Mr. Gavin Grant should also be recognized as he provided a steadying hand and gave me an outside perspective that I sorely needed. Words cannot fairly capture my appreciation for Jodie, Deb, and Gavin.

While all the people at Penguin have been fabulous, I must sincerely thank Mrs. Denise Silvestro, who spearheaded the publisher's acceptance of my manuscript. I am also equally indebted to Andie, Mrs. Adrienne Avila, who expertly walked me through the publication process, giving me feedback when it was most needed.

I would be remiss if I did not thank Mrs. Ellen Brooks for her help and enthusiasm during the book's earliest stages; Mrs. Sue McCloskey, who created the chapter titles, wrote most of chapter one, and rewrote my book proposal; Mrs. Priscilla C. Goodwin, M.S., R.D., LDN, dietitian, who gave added credibility; and finally, Mr. Scott Finkelstein for his help with an earlier version of the manuscript.

Introduction

When was the last time your doctor asked whether your bowel movement left your bathroom smelling less than pleasant? Never, right?

This question and its answer are critical to understanding how to manage your health. Nearly everyone seems to expect and accept that bowel movements should stink. Unfortunately, the idea that they shouldn't, and that perhaps this odor signifies a problem, generally comes as a surprise. Actually, the fact that I'm even bringing up bathroom odor is shocking, as it can be taboo. But it's time to get serious about our digestive health and start speaking more openly about bowel movements, as they are a strong indicator of our overall health.

Every time you go to a doctor's office, they take your blood pressure because they know it's a major indicator of your overall health. Few doctors, if any, however, make the connection between smelly bowel movements and gastrointestinal problems such as indigestion, gas, stomach pain, cramps, nausea, loss of appetite, bloating, heartburn, trouble swallowing, or even more serious illnesses such as acid reflux, irritable bowel syndrome (IBS), Crohn's disease, ulcerative colitis, and diverticulosis. With all of the medical advances we have made in the last few decades, it's hard to believe that close to eighty million people in the United States still live with these chronic and at times serious gastrointestinal conditions. Such illnesses, if and when they aren't properly treated, have a major impact on the overall health and the quality of people's lives.

It seems that if your doctor discovers that you have symptoms of any of these conditions, a raft of prescriptions are available to write. But unfortunately, all too often these drugs treat the symptoms, not the cause. Not only will you still have the underlying problem, but your digestive system, with the "help" of these drugs, may become even more incapable of functioning properly. Either that or you will feel better for a while on these prescription medicines, only to have your symptoms return some years later.

If only doctors would treat the problem! The problem underlying most gastrointestinal illnesses is none other than constipation, a commonly known but rarely recognized ailment that contributes to the prevalence of numerous and often severe illnesses. Even when it is recognized, this ailment is often not taken seriously, and popular remedies used to treat it often exacerbate rather than cure the underlying condition. However, many people have this ailment without even realizing it. Read that sentence again. It is the most important thing I have to tell you. Constipation is rampant all across the United States and is disrupting people's health in various ways, yet people aren't aware that they are constipated or that this is triggering other illnesses.

Even if your doctor asks you about your bowels when you report stomach problems (an amazing number of doctors never do), he or she is unlikely to ask about the odor and give you a diagnosis of constipation as a result of it. Even if you tell your doctor that you are having smelly bowel movements every day or every other day, your doctor will likely not discuss the possibility of constipation. Instead we are told that everyone is different; some people have two or three bowel movements a day and others two or three a week, and that's all right.

It is not all right.

Most people believe that they know what constipation is. Indeed, constipation is what we experience when our bowels don't move for days or even weeks at a time and when stools are hard and small. Although this is fact, this is not just *simple* constipation, but more *extreme* constipation. Unfortunately, this extreme constipation is generally the only type that people tend to recognize as such and the type that makes a doctor's radar screen. However, any bowel movement with a bad odor is a sign of constipation.

Why is this? A healthy digestive system moves its waste products out of the body within twenty-four hours of eating, before these "leftovers" have a chance to putrefy inside the gut. This means you should be having several significant bowel movements every day. If movements occur with less frequency than what your body needs, smells and problems can arise. I realize that nearly everyone is skeptical as they read these sentences, nonetheless, it is true. Would you willingly eat spoiled, rotting food? Of course not. But if your bowel movements have a foul odor, you are filled with food that has spoiled and decayed. Over time, this is wreaking enormous harm on your body. Think about it: With rotting food just sitting in your body and intestines all day, it shouldn't come as a surprise that you may experience stomach pain, gas, bloating, and acid indigestion. To compound the seriousness of this, these symptoms are sometimes harbingers of more serious health problems, and some evidence shows that many types of cancer and even Alzheimer's disease may be directly connected to constipation. I'm not trying to scare you, but I'm alerting you to a new reality.

Letting go of old notions and misconceptions regarding our digestion, specifically as it relates to constipation, is crucial in finding your way to better digestive and overall health. Knowledge of constipation has changed considerably since I first attended Duke University Medical School more than thirty years ago. Back then, ideas about bathroom habits were based on a British study published in 1965.[1] This study showed that 99 percent of "healthy individuals" moved their bowels as often as three times a day or as infrequently as twice weekly. Bowel habits that fell within this wide range were considered normal. More frequent stools were thought to represent diarrhea, especially if they were loose or watery. Less frequent bowel habits indicated constipation. More than 1 cup (200 g) of stool daily was also thought to represent diarrhea.

These conclusions have been etched in the minds of doctors ever since.

A 1987 study by Sandler and Drossman followed the bowel habits of young and otherwise healthy adults who had no medical complaints.[2] These researchers reported that a person could be constipated and yet still have regular bowel habits. "But how is this possible?" you may ask. Although the patients' bowels were moving regularly, they weren't emptying them entirely with each visit to the bathroom. The findings from this study eventually changed the attitudes of many physicians, and the definition of constipation was broadened to include such complaints as straining, hard and/or lumpy stools, a sense of incomplete stool evacuation, and even the need to manually assist with bowel movements. This study was built on an earlier worldwide survey of bowel habits during the late 1960s by Dr. Denis Burkitt, formerly an Irish missionary surgeon working in Uganda.[3] Based on his research, Burkitt concluded that passing up to several foot-long stools every day may be normal and that constipation likely was contributing to many of Western society's illnesses, including coronary artery disease, acid reflux problems, gallbladder disease, colon cancer, appendicitis, diverticulitis, hemorrhoids, and even varicose veins.[4] Indeed, C. Everett Koop, M.D., Sc.D., former U.S. surgeon general wrote in the preface of *Burkitt Cancer Fiber*:

> Denis Burkitt made discoveries that have affected millions and millions of people, especially those who sought control of their diet in line with preventive medicine. . . . He also helped society and the medical community to understand that dietary fiber deficiency is one of the primary causes of many diseases in the industrialized world."[5]

Burkitt was a surgeon who did research on fiber and bowel habits, and I am a gastrointestinal (GI) physician taking care of people with all sorts of GI problems, and yet curiously we both came to almost identical conclusions about normal bowel habits. My principal difference with Burkitt is that I say it *is normal* to pass several nonsmelly foot-long stools every day, whereas he said it *may be normal*. I think passing several nonsmelly foot-long stools every day is possible and normal because I've had patients achieve this.

I know you are probably struggling to accept my definition of constipation and regularity, but my years as a GI doctor have enlightened me on this topic. I recall receiving a diagnosis that I didn't think matched up with the symptoms. Almost twenty years ago I saw internist Dr. Steve Logue for a routine physical exam, and he suggested that my blood pressure (134/84) might be causing my frequent migraine headaches. This seemed a rather odd comment, because at that time 134/84 was considered in the high-normal range. Although I thought the suggestion was off base, I had not been happy with my blood pressure at this level. So I started lisinopril at his suggestion, and my headaches vanished. These days my numbers would be labeled "prehypertension," and an internist wouldn't think twice about prescribing medication. But this was almost twenty years ago. Like my internist, I have found that it is not always easy to convince my patients that they have a problem that's made itself known through atypical symptoms. Patients are often surprised when I point to a constipation problem when they're complaining of IBS, diarrhea, or acid reflux. But I have seen my patients' health improve as a result of diagnosing and curing their constipation. I believe that I am ahead of my time in this broad definition of constipation.

Treating the Problem

Constipation can build up over a day or a week or even years of poor food choices. The lower intestinal system has to deal with old stool (think poisonous waste by-products) and loses its ability to perform properly. For decades, homeopathic health practitioners have realized that we have this poison stored in our bodies, and they routinely recommend and perform high colonics to flush it out. Patients loved it, as afterward they would feel so much better, at least temporarily anyway. However, the poison returns the next day. This is because our intestinal system, plagued by years of unhealthy eating habits, is no longer working as it should. Also, colonics cannot wash the entire colon out, because they mostly reach only the left side. Basically, colonics are not natural! We weren't built to live this way! Right idea, wrong approach.

What's needed is a permanent cure for the constipation through revitalization of our gastrointestinal tract. My three-step fiber therapy program breaks new ground on our understanding as to how to use fiber supplements and laxatives. I have helped thousands of people with every imaginable digestive problem linked to constipation.

For some time now, *fiber* has been a magic word. I won't be the first to tell you that fiber is an essential component to good gastrointestinal health. Everyone talks about diets filled with fruits, vegetables, and whole grains. Your doctor may have prescribed a high-fiber (or even a low-fiber) diet or fiber supplements to help ease your symptoms. But the truth is more complex. If you've been constipated for months and years, eating more fruits, vegetables, and whole grains often simply won't work. For one thing, and this will probably surprise you, the fiber in fruits and vegetables and even most whole-grain breads and pastas does almost nothing for constipation. Even the laxative effect of prunes has little to do with their fiber content (more on this in Chapter 2).

The problem is that most doctors do not tell you which

type and how much fiber you should take, nor do they offer a structured program for you to follow that will enable you to measure your progress. Everyone knows that your doctor wants to check your blood pressure regularly when you take blood pressure medicines. But the corollary is not true: A high-fiber diet is frequently recommended, but no one talks about how the fiber should work with your system or the results you should expect to see, much less how to get there, and no one discusses what are the best foods and supplements and the amounts to use.

Many doctors and nutritionists fail to explain that for most of us, adding fiber willy-nilly often can do more harm than good. Our systems are already jammed up, and the wrong use of fiber can actually increase the constipation problem! So those of you who noticed that your morning dose of Metamucil or bran made you feel even more bloated were right after all.

Many people are surprised to learn that a healthy diet of fiber-rich foods often is not enough, and that there are good laxatives that help the intestinal tract and strengthen and tone the colon as well as other laxatives to be avoided. Twenty years ago, many laxatives had an ingredient called phenolphthalein, which worked as an irritant to the bowel, creating spasmodic contractions that helped elimination. However, patients who used laxatives containing this substance often became increasingly dependent on them to have any movement at all. Basically, their bowels lost the ability to move on their own without that stimulant. The medical term for laxative dependency is *cathartic colon*. However, I have also become convinced that certain laxatives, if used properly, can strengthen the colon, and other laxatives may undermine it. My plan kick-starts your path to a healthy and strong GI tract using a proper mix of fiber supplements with a round of the "good" laxatives (if necessary).

After years of punishing our GI system, we need a professional fiber therapy plan that's been tested on many patients and proven successful. This book is about what works and why it works. This book truly represents a paradigm shift in our thinking about fiber and bathroom habits. This book will improve your situation and likely cure your constipation.

How My Fiber Therapy Was Created

Over the years, I have worked with patients with all kinds of gastrointestinal issues, but it didn't take long for me to realize that the medications and other available treatments for GI issues were just not doing the job. I began to think that the key to managing gastrointestinal problems and relieving its symptoms might be as simple as doing a major cleaning out of the digestive system to rid it of years' worth of damage and buildup caused by inadequate bathroom habits and unintentional neglect of the GI tract.

My theory is that a long-term pattern of insufficient results in the bathroom causes the transit of undigested food through the intestines to slow down, which in turn leads to food decay in the gut, trapping gas and ultimately causing many GI conditions. The foundations for this theory began back in the mid-1980s, and one patient history particularly stands out (see page xx).

So I started experimenting with the one treatment option in which I saw some potential: fiber. Fiber use had long been touted as a method for managing gastrointestinal problems, but no one

FINDING THE FIRST PIECES OF THE PUZZLE

My patient was in his sixties and was having problems with diarrhea, gas, and reflux. After taking him off the usual foods such as milk, high-fructose sodas, and fruits such as apples and prunes and yet seeing no improvement, I suggested that he try taking Metamucil once a day, because he had offhandedly mentioned that the bathroom odor was particularly offensive. My hunch at the time was that by taking Metamucil regularly, the patient might have larger and more frequent stools, and his gas might move out of his system better.

A few days after he started the Metamucil, all of his intestinal complaints vanished. I should add that it was a bit of a stretch for him to even consider taking Metamucil, because he had diarrhea and a prior history of extensive colon surgery, with less than a foot of colon remaining! His improvement helped me begin to notice the relationship between bathroom odor, excess gas, diarrhea, and reflux. The first few pieces of the fiber puzzle were starting to fall into place.

had come up with a methodical program that was truly effective. I began by prescribing fiber supplements and high-fiber foods, and I told my patients that the goal of this program was to help them produce excellent bathroom results (more on this in Chapter 1). I tracked my patients closely and made some adjustments along the way. I increased the amount of fiber supplements they took and added laxatives until their bathroom goals had been reached. The results were dramatic. My patients' GI problems virtually disappeared, and they were happier and healthier than they had ever been. We were all thrilled until a few months later, when a number of my patients began experiencing symptoms again. I realized then that in order for my fiber therapy to achieve lasting success, it needed to be a lifelong program. I then created a second, modified fiber program for lifelong use to help them maintain their gastrointestinal health.

Since then I have cured people in their eighties who had stopped eating and given up hope of ever feeling healthy again and were just waiting to die. One elderly woman in her nineties had already picked out her pallbearers. I have cured people in their twenties, thirties, and forties who believed that their IBS or acid reflux was just due to stress. When the digestive system is healthy and relaxed, you can handle whatever pressures and problems come your way.

In the course of this book, I will let you know exactly what to expect day by day and week by week on my program. I will bring you to the point where your intestinal system is back on track and you can enjoy an amazing array of appetizing and natural foods. *This fiber program actually lets you expand your food choices, rather than restricting them!* I promise that most of you will find yourself feeling like a new person. If you have painful stomach problems, they will become more manageable, if not entirely disappear. If you take a slew of prescription medicines for your GI tract, you will throw most if not all of them away. Many of you will get back your energy and positive feeling about life, wiping out that general feeling of fatigue and sometimes even low-grade depression that may accompany undiagnosed constipation.

I have led thousands of patients through the program, and I can tell you that no matter what your gastrointestinal condition or symptoms, you will almost certainly see dramatic results after just a short while on fiber therapy. If you're dissatisfied with your current treatment regimen, if you are tired of the cocktail of prescription medicines for your GI tract that you imagine you will be taking for the rest of your life, or if you're simply looking for an effective way to manage your annoying or embarrassing GI symptoms, you've come to the right place.

Of course, I am the first person to admit that my three-step fiber program can't help everyone. My heart goes out to my patients whom I can't help, especially because I offered them hope and then I just couldn't deliver the goods. This may be due to prior radiation injury to the pelvis, narcotic dependency for chronic pain, the bushelful of medicines and vitamin supplements that some people take with the best of intentions, a bed-to-chair existence caused by severe arthritis or back problems, or irreparable harm from decades of a neglected GI tract and long-standing constipation. Recall that sometimes there is only so much a cardiologist can do for a bad heart short of a heart transplant. So although the three-step fiber therapy program will help most of you (and an estimated 90 percent of my patients), unfortunately there is no 100 percent guarantee. Recently I saw a man in his mid-sixties who had been treated by several stomach specialists over three decades for gas, constant regurgitation, and severe abdominal pain. He had tried numerous medications and even anti-reflux surgery, but all to no avail. Six weeks after his first visit to my office he was feeling "two hundred percent better." My primary caution is that you read the first two chapters of this book to better understand what I recommend and why, so that you will have a much better chance of not only succeeding with my three-step fiber program but staying on it for the rest of your life.

Notes

1. Connell AM, Hilton C, Irvine G, Lennard-Jones JE, Misie-wicz J. Variation of bowel habits in two population samples. *Br Med J.* November 1965;2:1095–1099.

2. Sandler RS, Drossman DA. Bowel habits in young adults not seeking health care. *Dig Dis Sci.* 1987;32:841–845. See also Locke GR III, Pemberton JH, Phillips SF. AGA technical review on constipation. *Gastroenterology.* 2000;119:1766–1778.

3. I was not directly aware of Dr. Denis Burkitt's research until I spoke with Dr. Henry Lesesne in May of 2004.

4. Nelson ER. *Burkitt Cancer Fiber.* Brushton, NY: TEACH Services, Inc.; 1998.

5. Ibid.

CHAPTER 1

Proving a Theory: Constipation Is the Culprit

Because I grew up as a math and science whiz kid in a three-generation household of engineers, these past thirty-five-plus years in medicine have been a giant field trip of sorts for me, as I am actually an engineer wearing a white coat and carrying a stethoscope. My father enjoyed saying that his Duke engineering degree really did not teach him how to do anything, but it did teach him how to think, and so he could figure out just about whatever he needed. Like most of my peers in medical school, I started out with the general notion that I would be a doctor one day and leave the work of scientific analysis to others. And for many of those years in medical school and subsequent private practice, I had not the slightest inkling that my engineering background would allow me to unlock some of the most fundamental truths concerning our health: that the widely unrecognized disorder of constipation is rampant across the United States, and it contributes to or causes a vast array of disparate illnesses. During all this

I was also designing a simple three-step fiber program for every-day use.

Among the illnesses Dr. Denis Burkitt ascribed to constipation and deficient dietary fiber intake were reflux and heart-burn problems, diverticulosis and diverticulitis, gallbladder disease, appendicitis, colon cancer, coronary artery disease, hemorrhoids, and varicose veins. To Burkitt's list I have added irritable bowel syndrome (IBS), abdominal gas issues, persistent and unexplained diarrhea, most of the common types of cancer, and even Alzheimer's disease (see Chapter 10).

The foundations of this book ride on the shoulders of Dr. Burkitt's landmark research on fiber and health almost four decades ago. Burkitt enjoyed showing a cartoon slide at his lectures featuring an ambulance sitting at the bottom of a high cliff waiting patiently for people to miss the sharp turn in the road because there was no guardrail. The ambulance would then whisk all the "victims" away to the hospital. The ambulance represented modern health care today in which preventive care (the guardrail) is practically missing. For GI health, the guardrail is a high-quality fiber program that can prevent or at least delay the onset of many of these illnesses. From Burkitt's perspective as well as my own, fiber is indeed a low-cost solution to prevent many expensive illnesses—as in the old saying, "An ounce of prevention is worth a pound of cure."

Don't get me wrong. Heredity (genes) and our environment are also important to our health, but for the most part, our genetic background cannot yet be changed. But constipation is much like high blood pressure and high cholesterol, cutting across broad swaths of the nation. The problem is that people who know that they are constipated are just the tip of the iceberg. Those who don't realize it are the submerged part of that iceberg. Yet the inexorable consequences of unrecognized and untreated constipation are taking a heavy toll on our health. (See pages 4–5.)

This was one of the many lessons that I was to learn from my patients: Start with just a small amount of fiber and step up the fiber dose slowly; another lesson was that there is a connection between gas issues and constipation. But an elderly farmer (see page 4) also taught me that sometimes it's best to improvise, to look at a problem from a different angle. In some ways, he knew his system better than I did, and he brought a little common sense to his treatment. But even after solving his problem, I had not yet fully made the connection between constipation and excess gas. And gas, I was to learn, is only one of a wide array of symptoms, many of them far from obvious, that may present themselves to a patient with constipation. It was some time before I got my next lesson from a patient, who got me thinking about what "normal" bowel habits should actually be. (See pages 6–7.)

However, once I began vocalizing this opinion, I became anxious. Why? Because I had been educated at Duke. I was trained in evidence-based medicine. This meant that research should support what one said. If not, then the statement was likely invalid. Doctors should have facts, not opinions. I did not have any authority to back up what I was saying.[1] So where did I get this notion about what constituted healthy bathroom habits? I had not read anything that supported what I had just told this middle-aged woman. I was afraid that someone from the department of gastroenterology at Duke was going to call me after seeing one of my patients and demand an explanation. After hearing me out, I feared they might say, "Well, Dr. Jones,

A PIG FARMER WITH GAS PROBLEMS

Within my first few months of private practice, a retired farmer came to see me. I clearly remember his complaints: "Doc, I've got the worst gas! I don't know what to do! My stomach stays swollen all the time, and that bathroom odor is plain terrible!" He was not eating or drinking any of the usual foods (milk products, high-fructose beverages such as beer and soda, high-sorbitol-containing fruits such as apples and prunes, beans, and raw vegetables) that might cause gas problems. And according to him, his bowels were regular. I was befuddled. I had just passed my boards in gastroenterology (the field that specializes in treating digestive problems), and I had spent two years specializing in treating digestive problems. I had attended hundreds of medical conferences. I had also read several textbooks in internal medicine and gastroenterology from cover to cover. I had reviewed hundreds, if not thousands, of medical articles, yet something as simple as the treatment of excessive gas had never been covered.

We did some X-ray and lab tests, including a colonoscopy (in which a TV camera is inserted into the rectum to examine the large intestine). Everything checked out okay. The only thing I could think to suggest to this farmer was to take some Metamucil. Like several other products aimed at moving things along—Konsyl, Fiberall, and Hydrocil, to name a few—Metamucil's basic ingredient is the husk of a psyllium plant. Generally, these products call for 1 teaspoon one to three times a day dissolved in a tall glass of water. One can also find psyllium in All-Bran, Fiber One, and a few other high-fiber cereals. At the time, I thought

that by taking Metamucil regularly, the farmer might have larger
and more frequent stools, and that his gas might move out of
his system better. Looking back, my training at Duke must have
convinced me of the importance of fiber in GI health. I say this
because when we had our formal welcoming cocktail party for
my first partner in 1988 (five years after starting private practice
in Fayetteville, North Carolina), the invitation had the following
notation: "Take the night off from fiber! Come to a low-fiber
affair!" And as people left to go home for the evening, I passed
out samples of Metamucil! Although it made for a jovial evening,
there was an underlying message as to how important fiber was
even during those early years of beginning my practice in gastro-
enterology more than two decades ago.

But I digress. Two months later, this same farmer returned,
and he said that his stomach was even more swollen than ever,
and that the Metamucil made his gas worse. I suggested that
he give the Metamucil a little more time to work because his
problem had been going on for several years. He did not return
to the office for a year or so. When the farmer did return, he told
me that after leaving my office on his last visit, he decided to
take just a little bit of that Metamucil every day. "Each week,
I took just a little more. It took a long time, but now I'm tak-
ing the Metamucil just the way you said I should. My gas and
bloating have practically disappeared." Thinking back on it,
this farmer must have raised pigs, because you can't change a
pig's diet too quickly; you have to introduce new foods sparingly
at first.

WHAT AM I TRYING TO ACHIEVE WITH FIBER?

One fateful day in the mid-1980s, Ms. L came into the office. She was a middle-aged woman who, like my farmer patient, had stomach pain and excess gas. She was already taking Metamucil but to no avail. When she saw that I was discouraged that Metamucil wasn't working for her as I had hoped, she leaned forward, wrinkled up her nose and asked, "Just what am I trying to achieve with fiber?"

I was taken aback. At that time, I recommended fiber to just about everyone. Her question was like asking, "What is blood pressure medicine supposed to do?" Lower blood pressure, of course. Or, "Why am I taking cholesterol medicine?" To lower cholesterol, of course. These are simplistic answers to both questions, and so what was the answer to her question? Just what is the fiber supposed to do? The question was so basic, yet so profound.

where did you read that? In which journal? At what conference?" The dreaded phone call never came.

And thus began the paradigm shift in my thinking about what normal bowel habits should be. For perhaps five years, extending into the early 1990s, I discreetly told my patients this vital message; I actually wrote down on a piece of paper for my patients: "You need to pass one to three foot-long stools daily." If you aren't passing this much, it then followed, you are constipated. As time passed, some patients returned, saying that they did not get any better. Yet they were following my recommendations. Others did well for a while, but their problems eventually returned. I began to wonder whether perhaps I had underestimated what normal bowel habits should be. Finally, in the early

Remember Bill Cosby asking, "Why do we have air?" His surprisingly simple explanation was, "To blow up volleyballs, of course." Just like the reasons why we take blood pressure medication or cholesterol medication, the answer to Ms. L's question was equally simple. Suddenly, I thought of that farmer and of what I had been edging toward with this idea of keeping his bowels moving. Next I remember my voice cracking a little. I declared with as much confidence as I could, "Ma'am, you need to have one to three foot-long stools every day. You should fill up the bottom of that toilet bowl at least once a day." There, I said it. I was finally voicing an opinion about something that had been lurking in my mind ever since seeing that farmer. Ms. L didn't quibble. She also seemed to think this was reasonable. If the fiber was not doing the job, I told her, she probably needed a little help from Milk of Magnesia or prune juice. And Ms. L got better.

1990s, I began recommending that my patients take the maximum dose of Metamucil recommended by the manufacturer: 1 rounded teaspoon three times daily (if not sugar free, take 1 rounded tablespoon three times daily). Their new goal was to have three to five foot-long stools every day, instead of one to three. About this time, I came to hold another unsupported view that I learned from my patients. As with my response to Ms. L's question, my patients brought me around to it.

I can't tell you how many times I heard a patient or a patient's spouse remark, "It smells like somebody died in there!" After a while I came to realize that GI problems, whatever they are, and bad odor just seemed to go hand in hand. One summer, years back in my practice and after returning from a trip to Bolivia, I developed a persistent bout of diarrhea that I just couldn't shake. My first thought was to send a stool specimen to the lab to check for parasites and bacteria. But then it dawned on me that if I had a serious intestinal infestation, my bathroom shouldn't smell like someone had just died in there. That meant I must be stopped up, and if so, then I really didn't have diarrhea after all.

So I put myself back on a high-fiber diet and bingo! The diarrhea vanished. And if a GI doctor can't tell the difference between real diarrhea and constipation masquerading as diarrhea, you haven't got a chance. I have discussed this observation with Dr. Martin Poleski, FRCP, FACP, at Duke and he emphatically agreed that odd as it may sound, diarrhea can often be a sign of constipation.

Putting all of these observations together, I began developing the foundation for my fiber program, and I concluded that if you aren't producing this level of output and especially if there is a strong odor, you are constipated. It doesn't matter what it looks like, or how often you make those stops in the restroom. You are constipated.

There was resistance to this kind of intense bathroom commitment. Women, and especially small older women, think they don't eat nearly enough to warrant such bountiful outcomes. To them I try to explain that up until one hundred years ago, our world was labor intensive. We didn't have cars, microwaves, fast food, electricity, or running water for that matter. Life was hard. You had to carry the water that you had drawn out of the well or from the nearby stream into the house. You had a garden that you spaded and weeded regularly; you chopped wood and carried it into the house; you hiked five, ten, or even twenty miles just to get to the store, to the doctor, or to church. You ate the food that you grew, the animals that you raised. Although people back then were smaller than we are, they worked their bodies hard. And they ate a lot more food just to maintain their weight.

Why do you think obesity is such a problem today? Part of it is due to the fact that we hardly move. But part of it, too, is that the foods we eat are heavily processed and loaded with calories; also, our colon was designed to process a lot more indigestible bulk fiber than our present diet of largely processed food affords us. One hundred years ago, we didn't have wheat bread like you buy today; it was the real-deal wheat bread: dry, gritty, grainy, and largely indigestible. Food back then had more in common with straw and hay than the white bread and refined rice that we eat today, and people had to eat a lot of it to maintain their weight because they worked hard all day long to prepare for the drought or famine that was almost certainly around the corner. Fruit and vegetables didn't keep well, and people ate what they could grow, in much larger quantities than we do today. Who had time to process flour and husk individual grains of rice?

Basically we were designed to eat and poop more like a cow than a cat! It doesn't matter what you think is normal for you; it matters how your gut was designed. Your GI tract will run smoothly if you acknowledge this fact and act on it. My program is designed to offset all those years and years of missing fiber, to get those atrophied guts working seamlessly again, to speed up your GI tract, and to rid you of your GI complaints forever.

As with my farmer and his gas, I realized with Mr. R (see page 10) that a person can be constipated and yet not associate

CONSTIPATED WITHOUT KNOWING IT?

Mr. R, a sixty-year-old gentleman, came into my office one day and told me that ever since undergoing a normally routine operation four months earlier, he had been unable to eat. By the time he arrived in my office he was no longer eating anything at all and had lost more than forty pounds. Mr. R was quite flabbergasted as to how he was even able to walk around. "Doc, you gotta help me. I don't know what's wrong with me. I'll do anything you say," he told me with much desperation in his voice. After questioning him further, I found that he lacked appetite because he constantly felt full. Fortunately, he had been able to drink enough to keep from getting dehydrated. Other than this, Mr. R had no other complaints.

I rolled up my sleeves and began questioning him about the more ticklish details of his existence. His bowels moved only once or twice weekly, he said, which, given that he was not really eating, didn't seem unusual. I sat back pondering his situation for a few moments. Suddenly a highly unconventional diagnosis popped into my head.

the symptoms with this condition. This is why constipation remains undetected by even the most astute physicians. People are often taken aback when I suggest that their problems are nothing more complicated than constipation. If I tell them that I think their constipation may be central to all of their GI complaints, they are often even more skeptical. Yet this is not rocket science. If you have air in your gas line, or if your gas line is completely blocked, everyone knows that your engine isn't going to run well, if at all. And it is not too far of a stretch to understand that excess gas and constipation must go hand in hand.

"Mr. R, it could be that the only problem you have is that you are constipated," I suggested, feeling as if I had just thrown myself out there.

Mr. R wasn't nearly as open to my tentative diagnosis as I had hoped. "Constipated?" he asked. "How could I be constipated if I'm not eating anything?"

"The gut is one long connected tube," I explained, "and when your bowels move too slowly, excess gas is produced and may get backed up. Perhaps this is why you feel full all the time." We ran all the usual tests to check for the more serious ailments, but he agreed to start the fiber program, much to my delight. "Don't delay and wait for the results of the tests," I told him. "If nothing else, you shouldn't experience any harm from kick-starting your bowels into moving more periodically. And I would be willing to bet that it will make you feel much better in the end."

Following my advice, Mr. R reported that just a few weeks later he told his wife to stop at Hardee's because he was feeling hungry. "I ate a big sausage biscuit! She was so surprised!"

Understanding Your Digestive System

The digestive tract is made up of several different organs—the mouth, pharynx (throat), esophagus (swallowing tube), stomach, small intestine, and large intestine—each of which performs a different task. The gastrointestinal tract is about thirty feet long (much of which is tightly packed coils) and travels from the mouth to the anus. Food is ingested at the beginning of the GI tract and processed as it moves through, and waste is propelled to the end of the tract and eliminated. When the process works as it should, it takes up to twenty-four hours to complete for each meal. If your GI tract is not working properly, it may take several days or even weeks for the "leftovers" to move through your GI tract.

The digestive process begins in your mouth when you chew food. A veritable cascade of enzymes and other substances begins to flood your upper digestive tract as the food travels through, starting with the salivary glands in your cheeks, under your jaw and under your tongue. When you swallow, your food is pushed down into the esophagus, which connects the throat above with the stomach below. At the junction of the esophagus and stomach, a circular muscle in your lower esophagus (called the lower esophageal sphincter) that works like a ringlike valve closing the passage between these two organs. However, as the food approaches this closed valve, the surrounding muscles relax just long enough to allow the food to pass into your stomach. When this valve fails to function properly, you have problems with acid reflux, heartburn, and such (more about this in Chapter 6). The food is then stored temporarily in your stomach.

The stomach, a large organ containing three layers of muscle, has four tasks to accomplish. First, the stomach must store the swallowed food and liquid. This requires the muscle of the upper part of the stomach to relax and accept large volumes of swallowed material. The second task is to mix up the food, liquid, and digestive juice produced by the stomach. The lower part of the stomach mixes these materials using wavelike muscle contractions called *peristalsis*. The third task is to acidify the food and liquid to kill any bacterial contamination. (Some studies suggest that people taking heartburn medications such as Nexium and Prilosec possibly have a slightly higher risk of pneumonia, bacterial overgrowth of the small intestine, and C. *difficile* colitis. This is because these medications prevent the stomach from making necessary acid, which in turn allows bacteria to colonize the upper intestinal tract and thereby are a potential cause of illness.) The fourth task of the stomach is to empty its contents slowly via the pylorus into the small intestine. The pylorus also contains a ringlike muscle that functions as the second major valve of the intestinal tract, which is designed to release small amounts of food and liquid out of the stomach over several hours.

The small intestine is where the most important stages of digestion and absorption occur. Food first travels through the duodenum, or the entrance to the small intestine, where a hormone called cholecystokinin (CCK) draws bile from the gallbladder to make fat more digestible. CCK also draws juices from the pancreas to lessen the acidity in the food mixture and additional enzymes that also help the digestion process. The pancreas has been called the "digestive gland" because its functioning is critical to healthy digestion. People with a sick pancreas (or chronic pancreatitis) can literally starve to death even though they are eating thousands of calories every day. As the food travels through the small intestine, these pancreatic enzymes and others break it down even further: Protein becomes amino acids, carbohydrates become simple sugars, and fat becomes glycerol and fatty acids. Only now can the nutrients and sugars be absorbed into the body. Villi, or the millions of tiny tonguelike projections that protrude from the small intestine's wall, pluck out the nutrients as they pass by and transfer them into the bloodstream. (Here's an interesting fact: It has been estimated that if you flattened out every single villus of the small intestine, the resulting surface area would be the size of a tennis court.)

Finally, after all possible nutrients have been absorbed through the walls of the small intestine, a mixture of undigested material, fiber, living and dead bacteria, and debris shed by the lining of the intestines is left over. This waste matter is propelled toward the large intestine, also known as the colon. As the waste moves through it, the colon absorbs water while forming stool. Muscle contractions in the colon push it toward the rectum. By the time it reaches the rectum, it is either solid, loose, or liquid, depending on how much water has been absorbed. The consistency of the stool is usually but not always related to how much time the food has spent in the GI tract.

What Contributes to Constipation?

Now that you can visualize how the digestive process works, let's talk about what causes constipation and how it can wreak havoc on the GI tract. Basically, constipation occurs when the colon absorbs too much water. This happens when the colon's muscle contractions become sluggish, causing stool to move through the colon too slowly. About 75 percent of normal stool consists of water, so when too much water is absorbed, the stool's consistency becomes hard and dry, and it is difficult (and often painful) to expel. When the "leftover" food waste is not propelled on through the GI tract in a timely fashion, the normal rhythm of GI peristalsis becomes interrupted, trapping gas, causing muscle spasms, and leading to reflux, nausea, pain, distention, and the like. In reality, the gut is one long tube. When one end becomes stopped up, everything can back up in the system. It's not complicated.

In terms of lifestyle, the most common cause of constipation is a lack of adequate amounts of quality fiber in the diet. Other contributing factors include lack of regular physical exercise, inadequate liquid intake, dieting, taking certain medications, and illnesses such as severe heart or kidney disease. Also, many occasional activities (as opposed to lifestyle choices) can cause constipation, such as sleeping later than usual, traveling by airplane, or taking an especially long road trip. The intestinal tract has a pacing system located in the upper stomach that behaves quite like a pacemaker. For instance, exercise and fever make the heart pacemaker fire more rapidly, and relaxation and sleep cause it to slow down. The stomach pacemaker runs at a much slower rate, about three cycles per minute. It is also affected by sleep, especially so that when you sleep later than usual your bathroom results slow down. Long sedentary trips cause pooling of blood in your legs due to inactivity, and this likely also contributes to impaired gut functioning. Understanding how your GI tract works and making proper use of fiber, exercise, and good laxatives when necessary is the key to both resolving constipation and managing your GI condition, and that's where my fiber therapy program comes in.

Signs That You Are Constipated

I hope that by now you have accepted the idea that constipation is much more than just an inability to have a bowel movement or straining to pass a hard stool, and other important symptoms are often overlooked. Because many if not most people with constipation don't exhibit the classic symptoms, in this section I will discuss each of these symptoms in detail and help you assess whether you are constipated.

If you have any of the following complaints on a regular basis, chances are good that you are constipated.

Bad Breath

Constipation-related bad breath is due to either bacterial overgrowth in the small bowel caused by a weak or incompetent ileocecal valve (the sphincter valve located where the large and small intestine meet), gas in the colon backing up through that same valve, or both. Another possible explanation is that you may be exhaling gas absorbed by your colon and produced by your bacterial flora. However, several patients have advised me that their halitosis vanished once excellent bowel habits were established. Of course, there are other causes of bad breath, such as poor dental hygiene.

Belching, Bloating, Breaking Wind, and Rumbling

These problems are all different ways that our bodies handle the same thing: excess gas. Gas problems most commonly happen when the "leftovers" (undigested food material) move too slowly through your digestive system, which is essentially the classic example of constipation. When the "leftovers" sit in your gut for long enough, they begin to decompose, creating gas waste that must be released at either the front or back end. Excess gas can also happen if your body is unable to digest certain complex sugars (more on all of this in Chapter 5).

Diarrhea

There are actually two types of diarrhea: acute and chronic. Acute diarrhea is a temporary condition (lasting usually a day or two and no longer than three weeks) that is often caused by a bacterial, viral, or parasitic infection but also may be an early sign of colitis. Signs of acute diarrhea include fever, weight loss, and blood in your stool. Contributing circumstances include international travel, a recent camping trip, well water exposure, and antibiotic use. Acute diarrhea rarely smells bad after the first couple of trips to the bathroom, when the colon has been purged of all the food that's been sitting there. I can well remember my three brothers and I having a severe bout of traveler's diarrhea when we were visiting Iran in the 1960s. We had one bathroom for the four of us. It seemed like every thirty minutes one of us was in there getting a workout. Yet oddly enough, there was almost no odor. The reason was that everything we had eaten had been flushed on through our GI tract soon after the illness began, and mostly what was running out of us was just watery material with almost no waste at all.

Chronic diarrhea, however, is a frequently unrecognized sign of constipation. It is often episodic and has a characteristically foul odor. Why would you have diarrhea on some days and not others if you had a physical problem such as colitis (an inflammatory condition of the colon)? Colitis doesn't come and go like that. Either you have colitis or you don't. Constipation certainly can. In my office, probably 90 percent (or more) of patients who complain of long-standing diarrhea are actually constipated. The remainder have some type of colitis or other problem like lactose or fructose intolerance (see Chapter 5). In this situation when constipation is masquerading as diarrhea, their diarrhea often comes and goes, and generally produces only small amounts of stool, or "a few squirts." Sometimes it may be more than that. Remember that my definition of normal bowel habits is several foot-long stools every day (this translates roughly into a quart — about one liter — or more of output), so when someone is putting out as much as a cup or so of watery stool a day and it mixes into the toilet water, it may look like a large amount. But if you measure what you are putting out, it is often surprisingly little.

Another way to assess your output is not to flush the toilet and let the residue settle. If not much settles at the bottom of the bowl, this is likely diarrhea due to constipation.

Another clue is excess gas. Food has to sit around long enough to spoil and produce that excess gas and bad odor. I will never forget Dr. Michael McLeod, a Duke professor, lecturing on diarrhea. He was discussing the seventy-two-hour stool collection that is sent to the lab and tested to analyze the severity of one's diarrhea. He used to say, "If they can't put it in the can, it isn't diarrhea!" How much on target he was. One easy way I convince my patients that constipation (and not diarrhea) is their problem is to suggest that they think of a fiber trial as a scientific test. If fiber makes your diarrhea better, then you are constipated. If the fiber makes your diarrhea worse, then you really do have true diarrhea, and more tests are necessary to determine the cause. If there is no change in your bowel habits (which happens occasionally), I suggest that the patient try stepping up the fiber dose to the full amount (see Chapter 3) and see what happens.

There is a long list of causes of diarrhea, and there is also a long list of lab tests that may need to be done to ascertain what may be causing your diarrhea. A fiber trial, on the other hand, is inexpensive and easy to do, and in my experience probably 90 percent of folks will learn that they are constipated. So why do a lot of expensive and potentially dangerous lab tests when the odds are that a simple, inexpensive fiber trial may diagnose and solve your problem? Of course, if constipation is indeed the culprit, remember that sometimes a tumor or even cancer can be causing it. Get yourself checked out either way, especially if you are forty or older, or if you are just not getting better after a couple of weeks or so of being on the fiber program.

Hard and Lumpy Stools

A healthy stool should be very soft and the texture should be similar to the consistency of cooked oatmeal that would collapse if it were not supported by the water in the toilet. This is because the food you eat has a high water content. If your "leftovers" are in and out of the body in twelve to twenty-four hours, the water content remains high, and so your stools should be very soft like cooked oatmeal. However, if your stools are hard and dry, this is a sign that whatever your GI complaint may be, constipation may be at the heart of your problem and an early harbinger of potential problems down the road. I learned early on that eating a large bowl of bran flakes prevented most of the misery of passing these hard stools. But as this book will show, a bowl of bran flakes is only a baby step in the right direction.

Hemorrhoids

When you spend too much time on the toilet trying to pass a stool, are constantly trying to pass one, or must strain very hard to pass one, you are exerting enormous pressure on your lower body's venous system. This can cause the veins in and around your anus to fill with blood and swell up, which creates painful hemorrhoids. (Not surprisingly, constipation is also one of the causes of varicose veins in your legs.)

Rectal Pain

The rectum is a muscle that allows us to pass stool and, like most other muscles, it needs to be stretched in order to work properly. If your stools are small, then your rectum never fully stretches as it should. Small stools also take a lot of effort to pass because it's harder for your body to expel them than to expel large bulky ones. All this effort can cause muscle spasms due to lack of proper stretching. The pain can be quite severe at times, even waking the individual at night. Sometimes it may feel like a hot poker in there. One related medical term for this condition is *proctalgia fugax*, procto means rectum, algia means pain and fugax means fleeting. For several years, a German woman would periodically rush into my office with excruciating rectal pain. She had tried sitz baths and suppositories without help. Once she had established excellent bowel habits by following the fiber program, her problem vanished entirely. Recently she came in for a follow-up visit, some ten years later. Her problem with the severe rectal pain had vanished.

Seepage

Seepage (when mucus and/or stool leaks through your anus) is an increasingly common problem for people as they age. Many people mistakenly assume that seepage is a natural aging process and that they should just deal with it. This isn't the way it has to be for most folks. Seepage usually occurs when the rectum does not stretch regularly with large, bulky stools as it should, causing the muscle to become spastic. A spastic rectum fails to properly accommodate stool when it arrives. A healthy rectum will distend, holding more and more waste as it arrives, much as the upper part of the stomach does when you eat a large meal (see the section titled "Understanding Your Digestive System" earlier in this chapter). This normal accommodation by a healthy rectum allows stool to be held for hours until a convenient time for elimination occurs. A spastic rectum, on the other hand, will not distend as it should, and it may even not be aware that waste is present. Instead of holding the stool until it's time to eliminate it, everything often just keeps on moving through your system, with little or no warning, leading to seepage or incontinence. If you read about incontinence, you will find it to be much more complicated than the preceding description. However, for most folks who have not had any apparent damage to their spinal cord (such as in a car accident) or pudendal nerve injury (for example, from traumatic childbirth or surgery), seepage and incontinence is often functional and will likely resolve with a proper fiber program (see also Chapter 3). This often applies also to those of you who have seepage following hemorrhoid and other types of rectal surgery. Your surgeon may even be convinced this is a problem you will have to live with for the rest of your life, but more often than not this is not the case, according to my patients. Further, many of my patients are mistakenly afraid of trying the fiber program since they have the fear that this will make their seepage worse. But how else will you know unless you try the fiber program?

Sense of Incomplete and Prolonged Evacuation
After a Bowel Movement

Many people also experience what's called *incomplete evacuation* and *prolonged evacuation*, which are some of the most common and well-known symptoms of constipation. Incomplete evacuation means that after a stool is passed, you have the sensation that not everything that needed to come out actually did so. Or you have to head right back to the bathroom to pass another small stool, sometimes within minutes of having just left the bathroom. Prolonged evacuation means that you feel like you have to move your bowels, but when you go to the bathroom, nothing much comes out or it takes several minutes or even longer for anything to pass. If you have this problem, you may find yourself returning to the bathroom over and over again through the course of a day, passing either very small stools or trying and failing, sometimes leaving you in severe discomfort, and it seems like you are spending more and more time in the bathroom. This usually occurs when you're passing too little to begin with. The rectum is designed to handle large bulky stools. When the system works as it should, the rectum receives a signal to have a bowel movement after it fills up. If you're not making enough waste (as most of us are not), after a while the rectum receives a signal to move everything along without being filled up, and the result is that it has to strain in order to squeeze out what little is in there. Try squeezing out toothpaste from a nearly empty tube; it takes a lot of work. To the contrary, normal bowel habits should be similar to squeezing out toothpaste effortlessly from a full tube, not an empty one.

Smelly Stools

It seems innocent enough, in fact downright thoughtful. Sometimes it's in the form of candles but usually a spray. It's the air freshener/deodorizer used to eliminate bad odors in the bathroom. Virtually no one realizes that it's a sign of disease. A healthy digestive system moves nonabsorbed food out of the body without odor—and it does so within twenty-four hours of ingesting it. Stool may retain the odor of the food you've eaten, but if so it should be faint and inoffensive, much like the odor you may notice when you walk into a grocery store. Food must rot in your digestive tract in order to create a foul smell, and this decomposition occurs when the leftovers that your body cannot digest and absorb stay in your body longer than they should. This rotting process has both short-term effects (such as gas and heartburn) and long-term effects (coronary artery disease, gallbladder disease, colon cancer, varicose veins and hemorrhoids, as well as quite possibly cancer and Alzheimer's disease) and can wreak havoc on your digestive tract and your health. Bad odor is one of the more reliable signs of constipation.

Straining During a Bowel Movement

Stools should be soft and easy to pass. You should be able to finish a bowel movement in less than one minute and effortlessly. If you're spending more than a few minutes on the toilet on a regular basis and especially if you frequently have to push to make something happen, this is a sign of constipation.

The Need for Manual Assistance During a Bowel Movement

Manual assistance during a bowel movement means that you literally use your hands to push the area around your anus, vagina, or abdominal area to help move your stool through. This often happens when people have small and/or hard stools to pass and is a sign of more severe constipation.

Unexplained Nausea with or Without Vomiting

When gas is trapped in the digestive tract, it can cause bowel distention, reflux, and/or heartburn. This in turn can cause some people to experience nausea, either with or without vomiting, which usually comes and goes. Of course, nausea can be a sign of many different problems, such as a sick gallbladder, but in my experience it is frequently a sign of unrecognized constipation. Remember that the gut is one long tube, and when the lower end of your gut (the colon) is not working as it should, then everything tends to back up in the system. This can lead to nausea, fullness, loss of appetite, and the like.

Unexplained Stomach Pain

Unexplained stomach pain is determined after you have been to a doctor and undergone all pertinent testing, and your pain is not caused by problems such as kidney stones, appendicitis, a stomach ulcer, or gallbladder disease. If you haven't seen a doctor yet, make an appointment today. It's important to identify or rule out other medical conditions that could be causing unexplained stomach pain. If you find yourself without such a diagnosis, then your stomach pain is probably caused by trapped gas and/or muscle spasms in your digestive tract.

Unexplained stomach pain is generally a long-term condition, and it often gets worse as the day progresses. It can last any-where from a few seconds to a few hours or longer, and it may be relieved if you lie down (gas can move more freely when you're lying down) or if you pass gas or stool. In such a situation, fiber therapy may just be what you have been looking for. (See also Chapter 5.)

Unexplained Weight Loss and Poor Appetite

When gas is trapped in your digestive system, it can affect your ability to eat. The trapped gas can make you feel so full that you have no appetite, leading to weight loss, as in Mr. R's case earlier in this chapter. You may not even be aware that you have a gas problem or a constipation problem. In my experience, constipation is much more commonly the cause of weight loss than more serious problems such as cancer or a sick gallblad-der. That said, you should still consider making an appoint-ment with your doctor to rule out the presence of these more serious conditions.

Urgent Need to Move Your Bowels

If you often feel a sudden and urgent need, as opposed to a gradually growing discomfort, this also can be a sign of con-stipation. This type of urgent need usually happens when your colon and rectum become brittle after years of small stools, which eventually leads to muscle spasms—your colon and rec-tum no longer have any flexibility, so when stools enter your rectum, you feel like you need to get rid of it right away. People interpret their urgency as a diarrhea problem, especially if their stools are loose or watery. But a healthy rectum will distend (like your stomach) and so urgency is actually another sign of constipation.

Fiber Therapy Can Reverse Damage Caused by Constipation

Regardless of how "obvious" your constipation problem is, rest assured that it is having a direct effect on your long-term health. Constipation causes three important things to happen. First, it slows the transit of food through your digestive system. As you now know, when food is not digested and expelled in a timely manner (within twenty-four hours), it begins to putrefy inside you. Second, constipation causes muscle spasms and gas to become trapped in your GI tract. These two elements are linked to the symptoms I discussed earlier and cause or contribute to almost every GI condition. Third, constipation allows chemicals and other toxic substances that are found in our diet and generated by the rotting process to build up and become highly concentrated. This means that the chemical content in the stool of a constipated person may be anywhere from ten to twenty times as concentrated as that of someone with large, bulky stools. Ultimately, these highly concentrated chemicals and toxins can be absorbed into the bloodstream and may lead to more serious, less treatable long-term health problems, such as coronary heart disease, gallbladder disease, and many types of cancer and Alzheimer's disease.

The good news is that my fiber therapy program, with its combination of fiber supplements, laxatives, and dietary fiber, will flush out your digestive tract, cleansing it of any leftover putrefied food, and help heal, or at least halt, the damage it has caused. This in turn will restore your digestive tract to a healthier state and alleviate your GI symptoms. The next chapter will give you the tools you need to put fiber therapy into action.

KEY POINTS TO REMEMBER

- You don't have to feel "constipated" to be constipated.

- A healthy GI tract should produce three to five (soft) non-smelly foot-long stools every day. This is roughly 1 quart of stool output daily.

- Just as a heart attack can present many different ways, so can constipation.

- Offensive odor almost always means constipation. It doesn't matter what your stool looks like.

- Weight loss, nausea, and poor appetite may be signs of constipation.

- Gas is a waste. When you are bloated, this means gas is trapped inside. Ergo, this is constipation; something is preventing the waste from making its way out.

- Most people with long-standing diarrhea probably have only constipation, and the diarrhea is just a by-product. Clues are odor, explosive stools, small amounts of sediment, excess gas, and intermittent diarrhea.

1. I was not directly aware of Dr. Denis Burkitt's research until I spoke with Dr. Henry Lesesne in May of 2004.

CHAPTER 2

Rethinking Sources of Fiber

Before I spell out the fiber program in detail (see Chapter 3), you will need to clearly understand several key concepts. Contrary to just about everything you have ever read, fruits, vegetables, and even whole-wheat or whole-grain breads and pastas are generally not a reliable source of good, high-quality fiber for maintenance of healthy bowel habits. By all means, eat your greens, vegetables, and whole grains for their nutritional value, but don't count on them generally to help your GI tract. High-fiber cereals and a few select whole-grain breads are where you will find the best sources of dietary fiber in addition to the fiber supplements.

The reason for this is that not all types of high-fiber foods and fiber supplements behave in your gut the same way. In fact, just rushing headlong into high-fiber foods or fiber supplements can often make matters worse. This chapter explains why this is so, and it will help you determine what types of fiber are best for you. Further, both the benefits and myths of laxatives are addressed, and I explain why certain laxatives can help strengthen and tone your colon. If, when, and how to use laxatives are also discussed in detail here. If you don't grasp these basic concepts of this chapter, then the fiber program won't make a whole lot of sense and you are less likely to make the lifestyle changes that I'm asking of you. I use case histories to illustrate these critical points so that you can more fully understand the rationale behind my recommendations.

Why Fruits, Vegetables, and Salads Are NOT Generally Good Sources of Fiber

Over the years, I have encountered probably a half dozen women in their twenties and thirties who have come into my office thinking that something must be wrong with their bodies. Each claimed to be feeling fine; it was just that each of them was moving their bowels only about once a month. I know that this sounds incredible, but yes, they indeed felt fine. Oddly enough, they also explained that they were eating fruits and vegetables basically every day. One thirty-two-year-old woman told me that she was following a "salad diet." She was eating two to three large bowls of salad every day in an attempt to lose weight. This woman became noticeably perturbed when I told her that she was actually far short of having enough good fiber in her diet and was stopped up as a result.

"How could I not be getting enough fiber? I just told you I was on a salad diet," the woman demanded.

"Salad does not contain the right type of fiber needed to keep your bowels healthy," I responded. The woman looked even more confused. I continued. "Fruits and vegetables contain a reasonable amount of soluble fiber, but that is not the kind of fiber you need. You want *insoluble* fiber. Insoluble fiber is essential for healthy bowel habits. This is what your diet is most definitely lacking."

In the end, after hearing the "fiber talk," this woman and other women like her agreed to try my treatment plan. Within only a few months, all began achieving excellent bathroom results. The key take-home message here is that even severe constipation can sometimes be well tolerated. This is what makes the disorder so difficult for most physicians to recognize and for patients to accept. The second key point is that many people, including dietitians and physicians, mistakenly believe that fruits and vegetables are a good source of fiber for the GI tract. This just isn't true. Even a dietitian like Priscilla Goodwin, MS, RD, LDN, who has now been a patient of mine for more than fifteen years, was initially hard to convince. But she finally came around, and she has been a vocal advocate of my fiber program, writing the following: "This is an outstanding collection of case stories that will benefit anyone who reads it."

So why are fruits and vegetables not a good source of dietary fiber for the GI tract? This is a hard question, and once again my response is predicated by what I have learned from my patients. First, what is fiber? Simply put, fiber is what plants are made of. There is no fiber in animal fats or meat. There are two types of fiber: soluble and insoluble. Insoluble fiber does not dissolve in water. Instead it avidly binds water, creating soft bulky stools that are easily passed through the intestines. Conversely, soluble fiber dissolves in water and is more likely to ferment in the large intestine. Therefore, soluble fiber has traditionally been thought to contribute less to GI health than insoluble fiber. However, soluble fiber has been shown to have other benefits, such as lowering your cholesterol level.

All of this sounds simple enough, but I'm surprised that fiber laxatives on the market often contain soluble fiber as their principal active ingredient. For instance, some of the newer fiber laxative supplements on the market include inulin (Fiber-Choice and Fibersure) as well as guar gum (EZ Fiber), and yet these fiber products contain principally soluble, not insoluble, fiber. In fact, in June 2007, noting how complicated and contradictory the literature is on dietary fiber, the British Nutrition Foundation stated that it is better to define fiber by what it does in the GI tract rather than by what it looks like chemically. In other words, we should focus on what fiber does to the body rather than what it looks like at the molecular level—to which I couldn't agree more.

So what's the deal? As best I can tell, the distinctions drawn on the labels between soluble and insoluble fiber are arbitrary, and their differences are defined more by what happens in a lab somewhere rather than what really happens in your body. Another possibility is that some manufacturers may tweak the labeling to make their products more appealing to the health-conscious public, because soluble fiber is thought to be heart healthy. Whatever the reason, I have found that labels can be misleading, and people shouldn't totally rely on what the label says. Also, I am convinced that insoluble fiber can ferment in your GI tract and this is why many people have gas complaints when eating a bran cereal or a psyllium product like Metamucil. What I am driving at is that it is far better to focus our attention on quality fiber products and foods that help your gut work as it was designed, rather than paying too much attention to the confusing jargon as to whether your fiber should be soluble or insoluble.

A major source of misinformation for the American public is the idea that high-fiber breads and pastas sold at your local grocery stores and bakeries contain good-quality fiber. Truth be told, over the years I have seldom encountered whole-wheat or whole-grain breads that worked well for the GI tract. One bread in particular to spotlight is Fiber Five (this bread is also sold by the trade name of "High Fiber 5 Bread"), manufactured by Great Harvest Bread Co. with stores across most of the U.S. Great Harvest Bread Co. is a "freedom franchise" company and as such there is no guarantee that your local Great Harvest store is making this bread. However, often their stores will start baking a bread in response to their customers' request. In fact, our local Great Harvest Bread store is now baking Fiber Five bread daily due to its demand, for which I take some credit. Oftentimes my patients have told me that they go to the Great Harvest store and just tell them they are my patient. Everybody who works there knows which bread I recommend. In Chapter 4, Fiber Five bread is described as the "real deal." In fact, it seemed that no matter how many slices of the other breads I ate, the Fiber Five always seemed to work much better. I was in a conundrum, because the fiber content in the Fiber Five bread was only slightly higher (5 g/slice) than the other whole-grain breads (3–4 g/slice) that they sold. At the time, this just did not make sense to me. In an e-mail communication with Bonnie Harry, Great Harvest Franchising Inc., I commented that I suspected that either something was taken out of the grain used to produce their other whole-grain breads, or else something was added to their Fiber Five. Ms. Harry advised me that nothing is removed from their whole-grain, whole-wheat breads, but flaxseed, oat bran, and wheat bran are *added* to Fiber Five bread to increase its fiber content.

I have found a second whole-grain bread that works as well as Fiber Five: *pan integral*, which is a generic whole-wheat bread sold by corner grocery stores everywhere in Bolivia. So the question arose: Why do the overwhelming majority of high-fiber breads sold in the United States appear to be in general a poor source of high-quality fiber (as far as the GI tract is concerned)? And why, in turn, are quality whole-wheat breads so easily found at your corner grocery store in Bolivia? It is possible that their whole grain breads produced by the corner bakery contain a good amount of what U.S. grain ·manufacturers would call "contaminants": the stems and stalks of the grain, which are neither nutritious nor particularly palatable. I thought that these so-called contaminants may be what make *pan integral* breads such high-quality fiber breads. And it would be logical to assume that the whole grain breads sold a century ago in the United States were produced using similar technology as is used today in Bolivia.

Ms. Harry at Great Harvest, however, suggested a second and more plausible explanation. There are many different types of grains, she said, and perhaps the grains used in Bolivia and a century ago in the United States were very different from what is used to produce whole-grain bread and pasta in the United States today. In fact, one encyclopedia reference stated that there are forty thousand different strains of wheat, and almost certainly the strains that are less palatable (and more likely to contain higher-quality insoluble fiber) have been superseded by more tasty grains, as the market is driven not by health, but by taste. Recall that for food in the United States, if it doesn't taste good, you are not going to buy it. Either way, unfortunately the American public has been lulled into thinking that whatever whole-wheat or whole-grain breads and pastas they buy today equate with a healthy high-fiber diet, when in reality nothing could be further from the truth.

Despite this, over the years innumerable patients, including the farmer whose story I shared in Chapter 1, have told me that "Metamucil hurts my stomach and gives me gas," or "Metamucil constipates me." If I believed what they were telling me, I had to ask myself, "Why would a laxative constipate or create gas?" Then it occurred to me that perhaps the fiber in Metamucil is only a very weak laxative and that people were more constipated than they realized. Rather than getting rid of their constipation, Metamucil was making it worse. If that was the case, I thought, then my patients needed to take stronger action. I advised my patients to take a laxative when they started the fiber program if they had much excess gas or obvious constipation; I also told those who had regular bowel habits that they would likely need to add a laxative such as Milk of Magnesia or MiraLax soon after starting the fiber program. So patients were told, "Metamucil and Citrucel stop you up because they are weak laxatives and not strong enough to do the job." The important message here is that not all fiber sources act the same way. As I've already shown, fruits and vegetables alone aren't a very good source of fiber for the GI tract. And for many of my patients, I learned that Metamucil and bran were too rough. I just didn't know better. Today

I discourage my patients from beginning with Metamucil or bran. Don't get me wrong; I think they are both a fabulous source of high-quality fiber, but I consider them as inappropriate as a ten-speed bicycle is for someone only just learning to ride a bike. You need to begin with training wheels. Only as you gain confidence and agility does it make sense for you to take up the ten-speed models. Far too often I have heard from my patients complaining about how much gas and cramps Metamucil and bran have caused them over the years. Many have said that there is no way in the world that they would ever try the stuff again. But now there is a much easier way for folks to get onto a good fiber program, and later eventually even enjoy bran and Metamucil.

Citrucel and Benefiber

In the mid 1980s, I attended a medical meeting in New Orleans. At one of the pharmaceutical booths, there was a large fountain that was flowing with an orange liquid with a sign that said "Citrucel." I only glanced at the booth, but my colleague Dr. Steve Logue picked up a few samples. At lunch that day, Steve pulled out the Citrucel and mixed it in two glasses of water. Steve was able to sweet-talk me into taking the stuff. He told me that we should think of this as a scientific experiment to see if it really was what it was cracked up to be. After lunch we drove to the airport to fly home. Meanwhile the Citrucel was quickly and quietly going about its business. When we got off the plane, both of us headed straight to the nearest men's restroom. Wonder of wonders, there were two vacant stalls, which we put to good use. We used phrases like "What was that stuff, dynamite?" and "We've got to buy stock in that company." (A disclaimer: I do not and I have not owned shares of stock in any pharmaceutical or fiber manufacturer.)

Soon I began enthusiastically recommending Citrucel. At first, most of my patients did wonderfully. Yet within a few months, most of their problems with the excess gas and pain eventually returned. I didn't understand it all back then, but this initial honeymoon phase everyone seemed to enjoy with Citrucel is crucial to understanding how to best introduce fiber into your diet.

Citrucel is an artificial type of fiber, a synthetic product—you take cellulose, which is a plant product, and then methylate it (a chemical reaction that alters the physical properties of cellulose), and voilà, you have Citrucel. GlaxoSmithKline actually had a patent on this product. So, because it is synthetic, not found in nature, this means that your gut has never been exposed to the stuff and lacks the bacteria that can break it down. It is literally indigestible. That is why, initially at least, Citrucel moves right on through you and doesn't cause much gas. However, if excellent bathroom habits are not quickly established after beginning Citrucel, as is the case for most folks, sooner or later your body becomes acclimated to Citrucel; the bacteria population needed to break it down establishes itself in your gut and gets to work fermenting it; and lo and behold, all your old gas and pain problems return. As best I can tell, this honeymoon phase with Citrucel lasts about six months, give or take a few months. So I tell my patients that they will do well on Citrucel for perhaps six months, but if they don't fully buy into the program and get the bathroom results that are needed, very likely all their problems will once again reappear.

This is why it is crucial to get all those "leftovers" out of your system as soon as possible. If we don't scour those pipes, all those hungry bacteria in your colon will begin a veritable feast on whatever fiber source you have selected and begin to fire up that fermentation process I discussed in Chapter 1. Once excess gas starts to get produced, a gas pocket can form anywhere in your GI tract. This in turn leads to air trapping, like air in your car's gas line. Once you get a gas pocket, everything slows down even more and you experience that familiar cramping pain and/or gas problem that brought you to this book in the first place. So although I don't generally recommend Citrucel long-term (because it is a synthetic product), it is an excellent first step to getting started on the fiber program.

Fortunately, there is now a second product on the market, Benefiber, which behaves a lot like Citrucel. Two natural products, wheat and dextrin (dextrin comes from starch), were combined to make wheat dextrin, which is Benefiber. Make no mistake: Although Benefiber contains only "natural products," as in Citrucel, they have been chemically altered. This is why Benefiber says on the label that it is essentially gluten free, when in reality wheat is loaded with gluten. To say that Benefiber has wheat and yet no gluten is almost a contradiction, unless one realizes that the wheat has been altered chemically in some manner. One of my colleagues a couple of years back commented that his patients were overall very pleased with Benefiber. My initial experience with Benefiber was also quite positive. Once again this was a honeymoon-type affair. Unless excellent bathroom stops were achieved, within a matter of months many of my patients were again experiencing all their abdominal pain and gas problems.

The point here is that either Citrucel or Benefiber is an excellent first choice to introduce fiber into your diet as painlessly as possible, beginning with small doses and working up toward larger ones. However, if you never commit to the fiber program goal, your problems with abdominal gas, reflux, IBS, and such almost certainly will return. I advocate using this honeymoon effect with Citrucel or Benefiber as the most painless way to get your GI tract moving as it should.

When you are working with a colon damaged by years of neglect, it will take a period of time before the full benefits of dietary fiber become apparent. Initially, your output will likely be subpar without a little extra help. This brings me to the second essential element of my fiber program. I had a friend who lived in a house with a basement. Like many basements it was dark and dank with a funny smell. And, like many people with basements, he didn't really want or need to spend much time down there. One day, however, he found he had to visit the basement for some reason or other, and this is how he discovered that his water pipe was broken and the entire basement was flooded. Even though life upstairs had continued as if nothing was wrong, the damage to the foundation of the house was extensive. So it is with the colon. If we wait decades before doing something about the fiber deficiency problem down there, there may be extensive damage before we realize anything is wrong. My friend was eventually able to repair the damage to his house, but at great cost. Similarly, repairing a gut often means first using the right kind of fiber product in combination with a good-quality laxative that will help strengthen and tone your system, before beginning the third and final stage of my program.

So, I repeat: Don't start out on the wrong kinds of fiber. Metamucil and bran are great for the GI tract and all, but I introduce those at the end of my fiber program. I recommend that you move over to bran and Metamucil only when you are making great bathroom stops with excellent output on a consis- tent basis, with or without the help of laxatives. Because I think Metamucil and bran are good products, I actually encourage my patients to do so, and they are definitely "more natural." But by the same token, if one of my patients calls and indicates that he or she is in trouble, I almost always have the patient go back to Benefiber or Citrucel: Let everything stabilize; get rid of that gas lock situation by using laxatives if needed. Once the dust has settled and everything is going the way it should, the patient can then move on.

Mr. A (see page 40) exemplifies this important concept concerning the management of constipation: The colon behaves much like a heavy railroad car. The railroad car is so heavy that it takes a powerful locomotive to get it rolling. Old-timers say that twenty or thirty men using ropes and pulleys can get a railroad car rolling on level tracks. However, once the inertia of the heavy railroad car is overcome, they say that just two or three men can keep it rolling down the tracks. With prolonged "vitamin F" (F for fiber) deficiency, the muscle of the colon becomes thickened (hypertrophied), and normal bowel hab- its can be quite difficult to achieve. At first glance, this would seem counterintuitive, but it is true. The same is also true for the heart. Long-standing, untreated high blood pressure

WHY SOME LAXATIVES CAN MAKE YOUR COLON STRONGER

Mr. A, an elderly gentleman of ninety with a significant hearing impairment, came into my office with his daughter for treatment. At each visit, he would shout, "All my life, I've been constipated! All my life, I've been constipated!" I can still hear him now, walking down the hall, booming out his complaint. Every time he walked into my office and before he sat down, over and over again with the exact same cadence and the exact same words, he would start this barrage of complaints. It seemed that ever since his toddler years, he had been constipated. Mr. A. said that he was now taking six Dulcolax (bisacodyl) tablets once weekly so that he could have a bowel movement that week, "if I'm lucky." Mr. R's physical exam was unremarkable, and his stool was negative for blood.

I told Mr. A that I was not certain I could help him, but I was willing to try. A lot depended on him, and I made this very clear to him and his daughter. I told Mr. A to start with a small amount of Metamucil twice daily and to take Milk of Magnesia as often as twice daily. I also told him to stop taking the Dulcolax tablets (today, I would have suggested that he taper off the laxative over a few months, rather than stopping it suddenly, and to start with Citrucel or Benefiber). For additional help, I suggested that he use 1 quart of lukewarm-water enemas as needed. (The best place to find enema bags is at the pharmacy. They are sold as a "douche bag enema" and cost around $30 to $40, but are reusable. Also make sure that you check the temperature of the water with your elbow before filling the bag.) I told Mr. A what I expected of him in the way of daily output. He was unfazed and completely motivated.

Mr. A's next several follow-up visits were notable for a lack of improvement. Despite daily enemas, he was unable to produce much of anything at all. We finally decided to replace the Milk of Magnesia with Colyte (polyethylene glycol—that big gallon jug many of you have drunk before having a colonoscopy). So on top of his-twice daily dose of Metamucil, he began drinking as much as 3–4 quarts of Colyte each day, followed by an enema if he failed to achieve good results in the bathroom. Actually, I advised Mr. A to use an enema after drinking one or two quarts of the Colyte, and if poor results, drink another one or two quarts and to repeat the enema if necessary. Finally, soon after beginning this modification of the program, Mr. A began having excellent bathroom stops, and he required fewer and fewer enemas. Over the next six months, Mr. A was also able to gradually wean off the Colyte, but he kept up with his twice-daily dose of Metamucil. So convinced was Mr. A of the importance of achieving his output goal that he built some type of contraption that allowed him to estimate more accurately how much he was actually passing. We joked about his getting a patent for this device. When I last saw Mr. A, he was only drinking a glass of prune juice each day plus taking his Metamucil twice daily. He was no longer shouting as he walked down the hall to my office; instead, the last few times I saw him, he had a great big grin on his face.

causes the walls of the heart to become thickened (hypertrophied), and eventually heart failure results if the hypertension goes untreated. Fiber is a poor laxative when everything has shut down, or when the railroad car has become frozen to the tracks. The Colyte plus the tap-water enemas were the thirty men needed to start Mr. A's colon working again. However, please also make sure that you have first been checked out by your doctor to be certain you don't have a bowel obstruction problem. Although in my experience this is uncommon, nonetheless it does occur.

Enemas can be helpful in getting the colon rolling. The way I introduce the idea of using enemas to my patients is the comment, "You know, desperate people do desperate things. There is only so much pushing from above that you can do with laxatives, and right now they aren't working very well. I

A YOUNG SCHOOLTEACHER WITH SEVERE CONSTIPATION

A twenty-eight-year-old schoolteacher came to see me with tremendous nausea and reflux as well as severe constipation. She could take the fiber but could not tolerate any of the laxatives because of her severe nausea, and she wasn't getting any bathroom results to speak of. We finally decided that the best thing for her to do was to use the warm-water enemas daily, thinking that once her bowels opened up, her nausea would get better. The first two weeks, she wound up using close to twenty enemas, but the next two weeks, she only needed a half dozen or so, and soon thereafter she was able to stop the enemas entirely. All of her complaints resolved once her bowels opened up.

WHAT I LEARNED FROM A BUSINESSMAN ABOUT LAXATIVES

Mr. B was a twenty-seven-year-old area businessman with a very active lifestyle. Though he ran up to thirty miles a week, he had a history of constipation and reflux. One day in the office, he complained that he was unable to stop the Milk of Magnesia altogether. He was following the fiber program, but he continued having to take Milk of Magnesia as often as twice weekly, and he had been doing so for more than a year. Not being sure what else to recommend for his situation, I improvised and suggested that he try taking the Milk of Magnesia every day, only just a little less at a time once he began to see excellent bathroom results. And in a matter of weeks, he had been able to taper off the Milk of Magnesia entirely.

think it's time to consider pulling from below to get everything moving again." Although not everyone is willing to use enemas, many are receptive to the idea. Among those who do, often they are pleased with the results.

Although many people may not become dependent on laxatives, the preceding stories are not uncommon. Bear in mind, however, that the newer laxative pills available on the market today are thought to be "safer," but I still encounter an occasional patient with a dependency problem. Some currently still on the market include Ex-Lax, Correctol, Dulcolax, Herb-Lax, and Colon Cleanse. But overall, full-blown laxative dependency is much more uncommon today than it was just ten to fifteen years back, especially since phenolphthalein was removed as an active ingredient from many over-the-counter laxative preparations. However, I generally urge my patients to

A YOUNG WOMAN WITH LAXATIVE DEPENDENCY

Ms. Z, a twenty-eight-year-old woman, requested an urgent office visit for severe constipation. Two years earlier, after having a baby, she had begun taking an over-the-counter laxative preparation once a week for constipation—this was back during the years when many laxatives contained phenolphthalein. As the weeks and months passed, her constipation became a little worse, and so from time to time she would gradually increase the laxative dose. By the time of her office visit, she had taken eight laxative tablets that weekend, and yet still she had no results. She then knew she needed help. I recommended the fiber program, including Milk of Magnesia and warm-water enemas as needed. I remember telling her that it looked like it was going to take "everything but the kitchen sink" just to get her bowels moving again. When I last saw Ms. Z, she told me that she was having excellent bathroom stops every day and she was no longer taking any laxative at all other than the bran and Metamucil.

avoid laxative pills. The one exception here is magnesium tablets, though they are generally not as effective as liquid magnesium preparations such as Milk of Magnesia and magnesium citrate. Although you may get a bathroom stop with a pill, the gas does not seem to move through as well. Not until you have large bulky stools does the gas have a better chance of moving on down your pipes. Beware of the recently released prescription Amitiza (lubiprostone; I expect others may be released in the near future), which is a lot of hype over nothing as far as I am concerned. Its maker claims that Amitiza helps up to 70 percent of the people taking it to have a bowel movement at least *three times a week!* Notice that I want my patients to have at least *several bowel movements a day—and indeed my fiber program makes this possible.*

Eventually I expect that the pharmaceutical industry will learn that one can't use a chemical to solve what is essentially a mechanical problem (a stopped-up plumbing system). One of the central concepts in this chapter is that osmotic laxatives (magnesium products, MiraLax, lactulose, prune juice, and prunes) can strengthen and tone your colon. Osmotic laxatives are substances that are poorly absorbed and that can hold water in your gut, sometimes even pulling more water into your gut. So you know that has got to be more natural than taking a chemical substance that first must be absorbed into your body to make your bowels move. In this area of health, it is clear to me that pharmaceutical research is most certainly going in the wrong direction. In principle I have a hard time accepting that the latest chemical discovery is going to be a blockbuster cure-all for the gut. But the key to using the osmotic laxatives is to take them daily and to realize you will likely need to do so for several weeks, if not several months, as exemplified in the three case histories just discussed. Most everyone tries to stop their laxatives too quickly or else takes them only a few times a week as they are worried about becoming dependent on them. This just is not an issue with these types of laxatives.

At any rate, these good laxatives include sorbitol. This is not a fiber but a special kind of sugar and an ingredient in prunes, prune juice, and certain other fruits such as apples that cannot be readily absorbed, resulting in a laxative effect. Sorbitol can be fermented, and thus at times it may cause more gas. (This is discussed further in Chapter 5.) An inexpensive osmotic laxative is magnesium, which is in Milk of Magnesia, citrate of magnesia, and magnesium tablets. It works exactly the same way as sorbitol does in terms of laxation. Because it is a metal, magnesium is the one product that is not easily fermented by colonic bacterial flora, no matter how long you use it. As a result, it causes the least gas of all the osmotic laxatives. So because magnesium is inexpensive, causes minimal gas, is good for your bones, is an antacid, and can strengthen your GI tract if used correctly, magnesium products are among my preferred laxatives. (A small glass of grape juice often helps prevent the bad aftertaste from Milk of Magnesia, and my patients tell me that the wild cherry and mint-flavored Milk of Magnesia are "not bad").

One possible problem with taking Milk of Magnesia (or magnesium tablets) every day is magnesium toxicity, which is rare; however, patients with significant kidney damage should especially avoid it. Although over the years I have encountered a few patients with high magnesium levels (found via an inexpensive lab test), this is most uncommon and I have yet to see anyone with actual magnesium toxicity. So if you are concerned about having to take a lot of magnesium to get those good bathroom results, it is easy enough to have your doctor check your blood magnesium level to see where you stand. Whatever works for you is best. So if you don't get good results with one laxative, there's no point in beating a dead horse; try something else. And if all else fails, use enemas and perhaps ask your doctor whether taking a Colyte-like solution (like Mr. A earlier) may be right for you. Today I would use NuLytely, TriLyte or MoviPrep, which are more palatable than Colyte.

Lactulose and MiraLax/GlycoLax (polyethylene glycol) are commercially sold products that work in the same fashion as sorbitol and magnesium. MiraLax also seems to have a honeymoon effect similar to Citrucel and Benefiber, because it is a synthetic product. It is a little pricey, but overall a great addition to your choice of laxatives. Today MiraLax is sold over the counter, but sometimes you can get it by prescription and it does have a generic, GlycoLax. I am not fond of lactulose primarily because of the excess gas it causes, but if it works for you, then fine. Lactulose is sold by prescription only.

Until December 2008, oral Phospho-soda products were available over the counter as a laxative solution. However, in response to a boxed warning concerning acute kidney injury by the FDA, C.B. Fleet withdrew its over-the-counter oral Phospho-soda preparation and their website states that it is now only available by prescription. Phospho-soda products are still also sold as an enema preparation. The Fleet enema is small volume and so it often is not as effective as the warm-water enema. Basically a larger enema (such as the warm-water or tap-water enema) will go higher up in your colon and thus tends to be more effective. OsmoPrep (sodium phosphate) and Visicol (sodium phosphate) are laxative products sometimes used in colonoscopy preps. These medicines are very concentrated and therefore pull water into the colon and are relatively effective laxatives given before colonoscopy and other procedures, but it is not a good idea to use them as routine laxatives because they may drop your calcium level and cause dehydration. There are also rare reports of kidney damage with these products, and people with hypertension or diabetes especially should not use these products. For these reasons, I generally do not recommend OsmoPrep or Visicol as purgatives for my patients prior to having a colonoscopy.

Finally, there is a third type of enema, the soapsuds enema, which can cause an allergic reaction called *soapsuds colitis.* I have seen this unfortunate and thankfully uncommon reaction, and so I do not recommend the soapsuds enema for my patients.

With these provisos in mind, don't be afraid to do what it takes to get the bathroom stops you need to achieve (provided your doctor has excluded other serious problems). My concern with any of the laxative pills is that folks think they can solve a mechanical problem with a pill. If your toilet is stopped up, you don't just use Drāno; you get out the plunger, which works far better and is easier on the plumbing. For most people, the plunger will mean the liquid laxatives such as Milk of Magnesia and MiraLax and an occasional enema. Indeed, once you get that old heavy railroad car rolling down the tracks, so much less effort is required to keep it rolling, it is unbelievable. As with Mr. A and the others mentioned earlier, and for most folks, these laxatives often can be gradually reduced in amount and even discontinued entirely as long as excellent output is maintained. However, please be checked out by your doctor to be certain you don't have a bowel obstruction problem.

The Most Common Mistakes Made in Managing Constipation

When people first add fiber to their diets, they tend to make any one of several errors. Either they take not enough fiber, or they take too much. People who err on the cautious side often feel better for a while, but sooner or later they tend to get into trouble—this may not happen for months or a few years down the road. In this case, bad odor in the bathroom and inadequate output are the most reliable clues that there is a lurking problem. The other possibility for those who undershoot their fiber needs is that they become disillusioned with the fiber program because it doesn't seem to be working much at all (often because they don't take a laxative in addition to the fiber) or they can't get off the laxatives quickly enough. These individuals are just not engaging the fiber program aggressively enough to get their intended results or else forget that this is a process that requires several weeks and oftentimes months before their body is fully adjusted to the program.

At the other end of the spectrum, some individuals don't follow instructions and sometimes overdose with fiber. Or they rush into fiber, especially the wrong types, and as a result have a lot of problems with gas and cramps and get discouraged. Also, when too much fiber is consumed, water has a difficult time penetrating into the fiber mass. Much of the fiber remains dry, which can result in a fiber clog, which is as bad as it sounds. Some years back, I saw a fellow referred by the emergency room for stomach pain. He was convinced he had a gallbladder problem when in reality he was just overdosing on fiber—he was eating a very large bowl of All-Bran each morning plus taking a couple of tablespoons of sugar-free Metamucil! By my calculations, he was getting about three times the recommended daily dose of fiber, and all of this was in the morning! Everything cleared up when he readjusted his fiber intake to a more reasonable level.

His case reminded me of an old cartoon of a doctor

examining a tree that seems to be planted in his patient's rear end. The caption reads, "This is a case of too much fiber!" So remember, if you get constipated, don't keep adding more and more fiber to your regimen. Instead, give your colon a gentle kick with a laxative such as Milk of Magnesia, MiraLax, prunes or prune juice, or even an enema or a glycerin suppository, and consider possibly cutting back on your dose of fiber for a while, or even switching to a different brand of fiber.

Then there are patients who are too cautious and do not take enough laxative to get the job done. I tell my patients that the worst thing to do is to take enough laxative to *almost* get results. It is better to overshoot, and then one can begin gradually cutting back on the laxative dose. Other patients try to stop the laxative too quickly, because they don't want to "get dependent on them." In my experience, dependency with the osmotic laxative class is just not a problem. Sometimes people find that they cannot reduce the laxative dose without getting into trouble. Usually this is because they have not taken the laxative daily, they never achieved the bathroom goal consistently, or else they didn't try to taper the dose off slowly.

Another error is that many folks just simply let their railroad car stop almost completely on the tracks before they begin to even think about doing something different. This is a big mistake. Be proactive! If you know from experience that everything is going to slow down, such as when you sleep in on the weekend or have a long road trip, don't wait for everything to shut down to make an adjustment. In the old days, it just wasn't a problem. Life was hard, and people ate plenty of food containing good-quality fiber. They also didn't have long road trips. Because their GI tract was so well toned, if there was any problem at all, they would eat a few prunes or an apple, and then their guts would resume the normal pace—hence the old saying, "An apple a day keeps the doctor away." In the twenty-first century people sleep in and travel a hundred miles or more at the drop of a hat. We don't eat as much food, trying to keep our weight down because we don't do as much physical labor as our bodies were designed to do. All of this contributes to constipation, whether we realize that we have a problem or not. When I sleep in on the weekend or when I go on a long road trip, I don't sit around and hope I get lucky that day or the next; instead I make an adjustment. Don't wait for the air-lock to set in and cause all kinds of mischief! Why should you wait for your bowels to shut down completely before making a change to your routine, even if it means just an extra prophy-lactic dose of prunes or Milk of Magnesia?

And keep a generous stock of Metamucil, Benefiber, and bran (or your preferred fiber) so that you won't be caught short. We typically keep five boxes of All-Bran (Bran Buds) at home, because it is our favorite high-fiber cereal. We keep an extra can of Metamucil and Benefiber for the same reason. Some years back, we got down to our last All-Bran box, and my wife, Lucy, complained that Harris Teeter had been out of them for more than a week. As it happened, I was in Raleigh that Sat-urday, and spotting a Harris Teeter, I went in and found nine boxes that I picked up. Lucy in the meantime made another trip to our Harris Teeter in Fayetteville just as a new cereal shipment arrived. She also brought home seven boxes. I think the stock of All-Bran probably jumped a quarter that day!

KEY POINTS TO REMEMBER

- Fruits and vegetables do not have much healthy fiber for regularity. The important thing is to consume good-quality fiber and to get results!

- I don't recommend more fiber than what dietitians and manufacturers recommend. The difference is that I tell you what that means in the bathroom, and how to get there, and why it is so important.

- Most "high-fiber" whole-wheat and whole-grain breads and pastas sold in the United States are not a good source of high-quality fiber from the gut's viewpoint. There are a few exceptions, such as Fiber Five bread sold by Great Harvest Bread Co.

- Not all types of fiber behave the same way in your gut. This book will help you select the fiber that will work best for you.

- Benefiber and Citrucel are synthetic fiber products. While they contain natural ingredients, they have been chemically altered. This gives these products a leg up on the competition, allowing you to start the fiber therapy program with less gas and cramps. But this is only a temporary effect, lasting about six months if excellent bowel habits are never established.

- Fiber foods and fiber supplements are very weak laxatives. They are great to maintain excellent bowel habits, but daily laxatives are often required to allow your GI tract to accept the fiber.

- There are basically two types of laxatives. Irritants may occasionally cause dependency (such as with Ex-Lax, Herb-Lax, Colon Cleanse, Dulcolax, and Correctol). However, dependency due to these types of laxatives is much less a problem today than only a decade ago.

- Osmotic laxatives (Milk of Magnesia, magnesium tablets, prunes, prune juice, apples, MiraLax, GlycoLax) are the good guys that can actually strengthen and tone your colon (in my opinion). These types of laxatives work best if taken DAILY, and you should only taper off slowly as long as consistent, excellent bowel habits are maintained.

- The colon often needs a strong initial push. Once it is moving, less intervention is needed. Your body's adaptation to laxatives is a process that usually takes weeks and often several months, or even possibly longer.

- Be proactive! Don't give your bowels an inch! Your grandmother really knew what she was talking about. If you know your bowels are going to slow down, such as when you are sleeping in on the weekend or taking a long trip, start a laxative or step up your laxative dose. Why wait for everything to shut down? It is much harder to get your GI tract back on track if you do.

- For the cost conscious, there are now generic alternatives available for Benefiber, Citrucel, and MiraLax.

CHAPTER 3

The Fiber Therapy Program

n 1980, I assembled my first baby carriage. Like most men, I put the directions aside and went right to work. When I found several leftover parts that looked like they belonged on the carriage, not on the floor, I read the directions. The fiber therapy program is the heart of this book, and this chapter is like the directions for assembling that baby carriage—and you don't really know what you are doing unless you have read the first two chapters of this book. This is the "how to" chapter, without much detailed explanation. Most folks just rush into fiber, not really understanding what they are doing, and then they think that fiber just doesn't work for them either because it causes too much gas or pain or because nothing much happens in the bathroom as they thought it should. This is much like my attempting to assemble that baby carriage; it is best to follow directions.

I enjoy telling my patients in the office, "One hat fits everybody!" Basically this means that I recommend the fiber therapy program for just about anyone who comes to see me in the office for whatever complaint they have, old or young, bowel resection or not, Crohn's disease or ulcerative colitis or not. Even if you come in for a colon cancer screening exam and have no complaints whatsoever, or if you have a liver problem, I will still slip in my "fiber talk" sometime during our conversation. The fiber therapy program is good for your general health. Certainly if I am looking at someone who I suspect has cancer, I will not advise starting the fiber program until we check the patient out, but even in that circumstance I mention it, saying that if everything checks out okay, it may be just what he or she needs.

Although the fiber therapy program works for almost everybody, like everything else you read, there are always disclaimers and exceptions. With folks over eighty who are also doing reasonably well, I mention the fiber program, but don't push it. I figure that if they have gotten that far without issues, no need to rock the boat. But if you are having GI issues, whether diverticulitis, gas issues, significant reflux problems, seepage problems, or whatever, I will generally nudge you to get on the program, even if you are ninety years old.

Also, if you have any special health situation, you should discuss it with your doctor or other health care provider before embarking on this program. I highlight several types of folks for whom this program is probably not a good idea, but unfortunately it is an incomplete list. I just cannot anticipate every exception. Rather I paint a broad picture of people who may wish to demur on following the fiber therapy program. Paraplegics and others with significant nerve injury to the pelvis, such as from radiation or pelvic trauma from a car accident, are often not good candidates for success with this program. This also includes women who have had pudendal nerve injury and/or major laceration of the pelvic floor related to childbirth. The central reason is that most of these people have bowel control issues (due to nerve damage, which a fiber program cannot fix), and more frequent bathroom stops is a negative for them. However, recall that people with bowel control issues who have no obvious reason for this problem often do very well and achieve bowel control with the fiber therapy program (see Chapter 1). Others who should probably not consider this program are people with poor general health, such as those with advanced Alzheimer's disease, people who have had a major stroke, and people who have mobility problems or general frailty from advanced cancer. To this list, many physicians would also add patients with recurrent bowel obstruction and people with diabetes who have severe stomach emptying problems (diabetic gastroparesis). Also, people who take narcotics regularly tend not to respond well to the program, generally because of narcotics' well-known constipating effects.

A few more key points before you start the fiber therapy program. Use only the synthetic fiber products I suggest. I cannot stress this enough. Don't use a different product just because it tastes good or because it claims to be as effective as everything else out on the market. Remember that each of the synthetic fiber products (Benefiber, Citrucel, and EZ Fiber) has a honeymoon effect (see Chapter 2). This means that they cause less gas and cramps for the first six months or so after you start using them. After that, gas, reflux and stomach cramps may be a problem if you chose not to heed my advice of achieving three to five foot-long stools daily, roughly 1 quart of stool or more each day. The other stipulation is that there should be minimal odor when passing stools or gas. Also, if you are eating a high-fiber cereal or oatmeal for breakfast and you are doing well, still start at Week 1, but just have the fiber supplement after supper and continue your bran cereal, shredded wheat, or oatmeal each morning. On the other hand, if you are having a cup or more of All-Bran or Fiber One cereal or if you are taking 1 heaping tablespoon of sugar-free Metamucil every day, and if you are doing well, then it is reasonable for you to skip Steps 1 and 2 and go right to Step 3. But please don't forget to take a laxative if you are not getting those excellent bathroom results.

Remember, many cereals such as Cheerios, Corn Flakes, Wheaties, and Total do not really have much fiber, and if you are having one of these cereals, you should take the fiber supplement twice daily. Also, on days when you don't have your high fiber cereal or oatmeal, take the fiber supplement twice that day. If you are having many gas problems, reflux issues, stomach cramps, or a lot of constipation issues, stop having your high-fiber cereal or oatmeal entirely and just take the fiber supplement *twice* each day. However, you quite likely would be happier starting at Week 2 or Week 3 of Step 1 of the fiber program.

Finally, if you know you are constipated, or if you have a lot of bloating and reflux problems, starting a laxative early would likely be wise. One more absolutely important piece of advice is to leave your fiber container out on the countertop in the kitchen, and even better, leave a second can out in your bathroom. We are creatures of habit and we need visual reminders to prompt us to do what we know we need to do. Learning to do anything twice daily is actually pretty difficult for most folks.

In the old days it was not a problem; all of our flour products were loaded with fiber. Because flour was cheap and most people had limited finances, everybody ate healthy servings of fiber daily. Not so today. We have to be intentional about what we are doing. Also, consider keeping an extra container of your preferred fiber product and cereal in your pantry. The fiber supplements should be on your packing list when you go out of town—but rather than taking the whole can, I use a resealable bag to take mine (and my fiber cereal for that matter).

So at long last, here is my three-step fiber program:

STEP 1

WEEK 1

Start with ½ tablespoon of Benefiber, Citrucel (sugar free), or EZ Fiber _twice_ daily, OR

Start with 1 Benefiber caplet or 1 Citrucel capsule _twice_ daily.

If one fiber supplement causes excess gas or cramps, try a different fiber product. Also, please note that if you have heartburn and reflux, the orange flavoring in the Citrucel powder may aggravate it.

During Week 1 of the program, most patients should have one stool daily, perhaps 6–10 inches long, or perhaps two smaller stools each day. If not, or if the stools are very small (only a couple of inches long each day), I suggest you take 1–4 tablespoons of Milk of Magnesia OR magnesium tablets (500–1,500 mg daily) along with the fiber supplement. This is not an either/or proposition. Take the laxative (if you need it) AND the fiber every day. You may use MiraLax, GlycoLax, prunes, apples, or their juices instead. Recall that Milk of Magnesia is an antacid and it helps your gas move through your system, plus it is inexpensive and good for your bones. Patients with kidney failure, however, should not use this product. MiraLax and GlycoLax are great products, but they are more expensive. Fruits such as apples and prunes and their juices cause more gas, but if this is not a problem for you, they are excellent to use.

If you have the dribbles, tiny little balls of stool, or a few squirts off and on all day long, this is also constipation (remember that diarrhea is a large amount of liquid stool), and starting a laxative, increasing the laxative dose, or even using a glycerin suppository or a warm-water enema may help empty everything out so that you get started moving as you should. Please recall that an occasional Fleet enema is fine, but if you use them daily, your calcium level possibly may drop. Warm-water enemas (use your elbow to check the water temperature) are safe even if used daily. As discussed earlier, I also don't recommend soapsuds enemas, as these may cause a colitis-type of problem (colitis is an inflamed large intestine).

Pretty much everything else to eat is fair game. The exception would be foods that contribute to acid reflux (especially if you have an acid reflux problem): Acidic foods such as orange juice, grapefruit juice, and tomato products. Caffeine, chocolate, mints and mint-flavored gum, alcohol, and most carbonated beverages may also exacerbate reflux. As will be discussed in Chapter 5, many people have problems with raw vegetables (such as cabbage, collards, broccoli, and lettuce) and legumes, but once you are achieving excellent bathroom results, these foods are generally well tolerated. So when asked, I tell my patients that their list of foods that they thought they couldn't eat are now fair game once they are well adjusted to the proper high-fiber program.

WEEK 2

> Take ¾ tablespoon of Benefiber, Citrucel (sugar free), or EZ
> Fiber <u>twice</u> daily, OR
>
> Take 2 Benefiber caplets or 2 Citrucel capsules <u>twice</u> daily.

Don't be surprised if the fiber feels like it is "constipating" you. Why is this? Why would a laxative constipate? It is because you were much more stopped up in the first place and you didn't even know that you had a problem (see Chapter 2). Don't be surprised at this or even concerned. Remember that fiber is a weak laxative and if your GI tract is sluggish to begin with, it often will not respond to the fiber as you would hope. In fact, I should note that probably one-third to one-half of the patients I've worked with did need to start a laxative by Week 2 of the program even if they said that they had regular bowel habits each day when I first saw them in the office. During Week 2, you should note that you are now going to the bathroom at least once and sometimes even twice a day with one foot-long stool each day or possibly even a little more. This may be two or three smaller six-inch stools each day. If this is not happening, you should start a laxative, increase the laxative dose, or even use a little help with a glycerin suppository or an enema. Remember, and this is key to the whole program, stay on top of your bowels! Don't back off. Your colon has been lackadaisical for years, and only now are you trying to do something about the problem. If you let a muscle cramp go for months and months (years for that matter), it is going to take some work to get that muscle back up to snuff—and this is not something you do twice a week; you know you have to work with that muscle every day. So it is with your colon. Take the laxative *every day*; don't be afraid. Laxative dependency is not a problem with the osmotic laxatives such as Milk of Magnesia, MiraLax, GlycoLax, prunes, apples, and their juices; indeed, these laxatives can make your colon stronger, but they work best only if you take them every day. I cannot stress enough this idea of taking your laxative daily (if you need it). When it comes to laxatives and enemas, my patients are like these young children, afraid to take their necessary laxative when I know how much it will help. The difference here is that most cuts in children will heal anyway by themselves, but in adults, constipation will not usually resolve by just taking fiber.

By now, your bathroom odor ought to be improving, and don't be surprised if you are starting to feel a little bit more energetic and even lighter on your feet. Why would this be? Getting all the leftovers out of your system before they have a chance to putrefy inside is the reason. This is not high-tech science. If you have had problems with gas, reflux, or pain, by now these often start to be either less intense, less frequent, or perhaps less prolonged. This is a process; don't expect to get well overnight. If your reflux, gas, or pain is getting worse during Week 2, and it is a problem, consider starting a laxative, stepping up the laxative dose, going back to Week 1 of Step 1, or as a last resort switching to one of the other fiber products listed earlier. Sometimes you also need to take an antacid such as Prilosec once or twice daily for the first few weeks (or longer) of the fiber program.

Of course, there may be setbacks along the way, especially if you like to sleep in on the weekend or go on long road trips, and this is particularly true for those of you with a severe spastic colon, such as irritable bowel syndrome or major reflux issues (see also Chapters 6 and 7). Also, if you have had significant GI issues for many years before starting this program, then it may

be a few weeks and possibly even longer before you begin reap-
ing the benefits. In this case, it may be better to stay on Week 2
one or two extra weeks before going forward and perhaps step
up your laxative dose to try to get your bowels moving as they
should. Listen to your gut. Back down on the fiber program,
even going all the way back to Week 1 of Step 1, if you are hav-
ing too much gas, reflux, or cramping. Once again, if needed,
use laxatives to help you achieve your goal of treatment; for
Week 2, this should be at least one foot-long stool every day or
two to three six-inch stools each day. Don't be afraid! Remem-
ber that laxatives such as Milk of Magnesia (MiraLax, Glyco-
Lax, magnesium tablets, prunes or apples, or their juices) and
even glycerin suppositories can make your colon stronger, but
these work best if you use them daily (see Chapter 2).

WEEK 3

Take 1 level tablespoon of Benefiber, Citrucel (sugar free), or
EZ Fiber <u>twice</u> daily, OR
Take 3 Benefiber caplets or 3 Citrucel capsules <u>twice</u> daily.

Only take this step if you have been getting good bathroom
results during Week 2 of the program. If not, then do another
week of Week 2. During Week 3 of the program, you should be
consistently having at least one and often two foot-long stools
each day, and your bathroom odor will be noticeably improved
from only a few weeks ago. If by now you have needed a laxa-
tive, you should continue it through this week and almost cer-
tainly the next several weeks of the fiber program. Again, don't
be alarmed. Most folks who need a laxative usually take it for
4–12 weeks, or possibly even longer. Instead, you should start

noticing how much better you feel as you get better results in the bathroom and how sluggish you feel on other days when this doesn't happen. Notice also that as time passes, your bathroom results improve, and also it takes less effort.

Most of us have been couch potatoes in our lives at one time or other (or indefinitely, for that matter!). Now you may think about getting back into shape by running a couple of miles a day. At first you will have to push yourself hard to get it done, and you will likely start by walking and running part of the way, but as you get more physically fit and your weight drops a little, you will eventually be able to almost coast while running the same distance. So it is with the large intestine. Remember that your colon is a muscle that takes time to get back in shape. It's really not much different from getting a couch potato back into shape. Be patient and learn to enjoy the ride.

WEEK 4

Take 1 slightly rounded tablespoon of Benefiber, Citrucel (sugar free), or EZ Fiber twice daily, OR

Take 4 Benefiber caplets or 4 Citrucel capsules twice daily.

If you read labels, you will have noticed that you are now taking the manufacturer's maximum recommended dose (and even a higher dose for capsules and caplets), and yet you are only on Week 4 of the program. Relax. Although my recommended doses of Citrucel, Benefiber, and EZ Fiber are different from those given by the manufacturer, my maximum twenty-four-hour fiber dose is basically the same. Research studies have shown that almost no one can do anything consistently three times a day every day. So the maximum twenty-four-hour dose of fiber that I recommend is the same as that recommended by the manufacturer; I just advise my patients to divide it in half rather than in thirds. For instance, for Benefiber caplets, the manufacturer's maximum dose is three caplets three times daily; this would be nine caplets of Benefiber in twenty-four hours. Notice that during Week 5 of the program (discussed shortly), I advise five Benefiber caplets twice daily—one caplet more than the manufacturer's recommendation every twenty-four hours. However, I use a different twenty-four-hour dose for the Citrucel capsules. This is because each Citrucel capsule contains only 0.5 g of methylcellulose. So twelve Citrucel capsules contain 6 g of methylcellulose, which is the same as the maximum recommended dose for the Citrucel powder—one scoop (2 g of methylcellulose) three times daily. However, be sure to drink a large glass of water to wash the pills/capsules down.

By now, bathroom odor should generally be a thing of the past, and your abdominal gas and bloating, stomach pain, and reflux should also have lessened, rather than being an everyday thing. If not, then you are not taking enough of the laxative or you have pushed too rapidly with the fiber. If you are feeling worse than when you started, try a different fiber product. Or consider going back to Week 1 of the program and starting over with a different fiber product, but being more aggressive with the laxatives. Admittedly, some people adapt much more slowly; if you are making progress in better bathroom results and reduced gas, pain, or reflux, that is much more important than the fact that all of your complaints have not yet completely vanished. During this week, you should be noting two and even occasionally three foot-long stools daily, or perhaps smaller stools but possibly four or five stools each day. Bad breath and headaches (if constipation related), seepage, noisy stomach, belching, excess gas, reflux, stomach pain, urgency, sense of incomplete evacuation, hemorrhoids, and irritable bowel all should be noticeably better or even absent. Your energy level should also be noticeably better.

WEEKS 5 AND 6

Take 1 heaping tablespoon of Benefiber, Citrucel (sugar free),
    or EZ Fiber twice daily, OR

Take 5 Benefiber caplets or 5 Citrucel capsules twice daily,
    and if you are on Citrucel capsules, then during Week 6 you
    should plan to take 6 capsules twice daily.

During Weeks 5 and 6, bathroom results should now be fabulous and you should be passing three foot-long stools every day, or perhaps a little less at a time but a bit more often. If your estimate is now 1 quart or more daily, your stools are very soft with minimal hints of bathroom odor, and this has all occurred over at least a week or longer, you can now try to reduce the laxative dose. Don't be surprised if your bathroom output drops and you have to step up the laxative dose once again. This is a process. It will take time, but eventually after a couple of weeks, or perhaps a couple of months, you will be able to reduce the laxative dose. Again, and I cannot stress this point too often, stay on top of your bowels! Milk of Magnesia and the other laxatives are your friend. They won't disappoint you, but you need to use them daily to get these results.

Now remember that the descriptions of Weeks 1 through 6 are rough guidelines only. Many folks will progress through the program more rapidly and do just fine. Others take longer, perhaps even three to four months, and some of you may take six to twelve months to get your bathroom results where they ought to be. Usually this is because you are being too cautious with the laxatives—not taking them daily or not taking enough (or not using an enema when necessary)—but sometimes it is because your large intestine muscles need more help. Wherever you fit into the schedule, the important thing is to be persistent, keep nudging your large intestines to do what you know they are supposed to do in the bathroom, and don't give in and settle for partial success. Listen to your body. It knows more than you think. This is extremely important.

Remember, don't stay indefinitely on Week 2 or Week 3 of the program. If you do so, your abdominal gas and reflux and/or pain problems will almost certainly return, and sooner than you think. These synthetic fiber products are artificial. That gives them a leg up on the competition such as Metamucil, Konsyl, and high-fiber cereals because the bacterial flora in your large intestine cannot recognize and ferment these synthetic fiber products as easily. But this phenomenon is only temporary. Eventually the bacterial flora in your large intestine will learn to recognize and ferment these products as if you were ingesting Metamucil or bran, and thus cause gas, pain, and reflux all over again. Getting everything moving along and out of the body in a timely fashion is the only long-term solution for reflux, abdominal gas, IBS (irritable bowel syndrome), and the like.

By now, many of you have already figured out that the amount of fiber I recommend is different than what is recommended by the manufacturer. This is because I have developed this concept of "fiber exchanges" instead of what the manufacturers recommend, which are "fiber servings." The difference between these two terms will be developed in Chapter 4. Ultimately, I expect that the manufacturers and the American Dietetic Association will embrace this idea of fiber exchanges and discard the term fiber servings to "level the playing ground" so that consumers will be able to easily interchange fiber products and high fiber foods by a quick glance at the label.

STEP 2

The heart of Step 1 is using the synthetic fiber products (which are generally so much easier on the gut), developing the habit of getting your fiber in twice daily, and, most important, achieving those excellent bowel habits daily that are so necessary for good health. When you are consistently achieving these results and after you have been on Week 5 (Week 6 if on the Citrucel capsules) for one or two weeks, you are now ready to move on to Step 2. Remember that you will generally stay on Step 1 for four to eight weeks before moving on to Step 2, which you will follow for one to two months, depending on your progress. Also, if you choose, you can stay on Week 5 or 6 of Step 1 or on Step 2 indefinitely. Just realize that Citrucel, Benefiber, and EZ Fiber are synthetic fiber products, and I suspect that their laxative effects, and possibly their health benefits, may not match the other "more natural" sources of fiber that will be used in Steps 2 and 3. I cannot stress enough the importance of getting those excellent bathroom results before moving to Step 2. The reason is that if you aren't, likely you will experience gas, cramps, or reflux problems because your gut is not ready to receive these more natural types of fiber products. It took me close to twenty years to figure this all out, so just trust my judgment if by now you still don't understand why this is so. Finally, those of you who were already eating a high-fiber cereal or oatmeal and continued it throughout Step 1 are now actually on Step 2! You can move on to Step 3 if you so choose. But know that you should go to Step 3 only if you are making those excellent bathroom stops.

Other clues that you are ready for Step 2 include minimal or no bathroom odor and no gas problems. In this step, your Benefiber or Citrucel dose is reduced to half of your daily dose, and you can now substitute another type of fiber. The idea here is to allow you the option to move to other types of fiber, but to make the transition slowly. Recall that bran and psyllium may cause gas and cramps. Therefore it is better to dip your toe in the water *first* before plunging into Step 3. Although this may seem confusing, the following sample menu should clarify this better.

Here are some menu examples for Week 1 of Step 2:

SAMPLE MENU FOR WEEK 1 OF STEP 2

DAY 1

MORNING:

   1 cup of Bran Flakes and 2 rounded teaspoons of Benefiber

EVENING:

   1 heaping tablespoon of Benefiber

DAY 2

MORNING:

   2 cups Shredded Wheat

EVENING:

   1 heaping tablespoon of Benefiber or EZ Fiber

DAY 3

MORNING:

1 cup oatmeal and 2 rounded teaspoons of Citrucel (sugar free)

EVENING:

1 heaping tablespoon of Citrucel (sugar free)

DAY 4

MORNING:

1 slice Fiber Five bread (Great Harvest Bread Co.) plus 2
    rounded teaspoons of Benefiber or EZ fiber

EVENING:

1 heaping tablespoon of Benefiber or EZ Fiber

DAY 5

MORNING:

1 cup Kashi Good Friends cereal

EVENING:

1 heaping tablespoon Citrucel (sugar free)

DAY 6

MORNING:

½ cup All-Bran Extra Fiber or Bran Buds for breakfast

EVENING:

1 heaping tablespoon of Benefiber

DAY 7

MORNING:

½ oup Fiber One

EVENING:

1 heaping tablespoon of Citrucel (sugar free)

While I am trying to be helpful with the preceding examples, it is important to recall that if you were using only Benefiber during Step 1, you should use only Benefiber during Step 2. The point is that it is best not to switch from one synthetic fiber to another day to day or even week to week. That way, if you have difficulty adjusting to the fiber program, or get into trouble a year later, you still have another synthetic fiber product to which your gut bacterial flora has not been exposed. Recall also that you have only about six months with Benefiber before the gas problems return—that is if you never get your bowel habits up to the necessary several large, soft foot-long stools daily. Remember also, your fiber should be continued twice daily. So on Step 2, you may choose to have 1 heaping tablespoon of Benefiber for the evening serving and take 2 teaspoons of Benefiber in the morning with a cup of oatmeal or bran flakes. If you are still getting excellent bathroom results, and you are still taking a laxative such as Milk of Magnesia, it is okay to drop the dose, but best to keep taking it daily. Remember that it is always best to wean off your laxative slowly but keep taking it every day (see Chapter 2). This is one of the more important aspects of Step 2 in the fiber therapy program: The more natural fibers found in high-quality fiber cereals and psyllium seem to have more potent laxative properties, which often allow you to more rapidly wean off the laxatives. But don't expect that just because you are on Step 2, you can stop your laxatives in a week. Look at what is happening. Reduce the laxative dose only if you continue to get excellent results. Remember to increase the laxative dose if your bathroom results are not what they should be or if you expect them to slow down because you are traveling or sleeping in that weekend. This is a process; it takes time. Everyone is different; go at your own pace, and you will be much happier if you do!

STEP 3

If you have done well with Step 2 for one or two months and are getting the required bathroom results, then it is now okay to move on to Step 3. The opposite is also true: If you are not passing several large, soft stools daily and if gas and odor are still a problem, you are not ready for Step 3. Rather, it would be a good idea to stay on Step 2 and perhaps to start a laxative (or increase the dose if you are already on a laxative) for a few weeks before moving to Step 3. Remember, it is also perfectly okay to stay on Step 1 or Step 2 indefinitely if you choose and if you are doing well. In Step 3, you can pretty much mix and match. But never take your eyes off your goal.

During this final step, the synthetic fiber products (Benefiber, Citrucel, and EZ Fiber) are stopped and you can now solely use other "more natural" fiber sources—high-fiber cereals, good-quality whole-grain breads (but remember that in my opinion, most whole-wheat and whole-grain breads and pastas sold in the United States are not a good source of high quality fiber), and psyllium products (Metamucil, Hydrocil, Konsyl, and Fiberall) as well as inulin products (Fibersure, FiberChoice) and others (see Chapter 4, as my recommended dose often varies from the manufacturer's recommendation for each product). Some people have no problem skipping Steps 1 and 2 and go right to Step 3 of the fiber program. This is great if you can do it, but I urge most people to follow the three-step program. Remember that if you are having GI issues while eating your favorite cereal or oatmeal, it is best for you to stop it entirely and take just Benefiber or Citrucel twice daily, that is, go back to Step 1 of the program.

During Step 3, you will find that it is easier to taper off the laxatives (if you are using them) because these products are generally more effective than Benefiber and Citrucel. Do *not* go cold turkey off laxatives. I cannot stress this enough. Typically it takes weeks, if not several months or longer, to get off the laxative. The older you are, the less active you are, the longer the problem has been around, the more medicines you take, the longer it takes to get off the laxative. There is no way around this. You have to be patient. Let your bathroom results tell you when it is time, and don't stop any earlier. Even younger people sometimes need several months or longer on the laxatives for their GI tract to adjust. Part of this is probably because younger people tend to travel a lot more, and they often have a more erratic schedule, such as sleeping in long hours on weekends and the like. Listen to your body. Be patient. It is better to focus your attention on the progress you are making, the fact that you are getting better and better bathroom results, than on quitting the laxatives. With time you will find that you need less effort to get those results. The laxatives and fiber are indeed doing the job of making your colon stronger as promised, but it is a slow process. Let me give you an example. Last year my back went out. I saw a chiropractor who suggested that I begin Pilates and regular massages in addition to my daily yoga. It has taken my back eight months to see the full benefits from these recommendations. So it is with your gut.

The key to Step 3 is consistently maintaining excellent bathroom results while you are moving to other fiber sources. Sometimes patients get far into the program but then suffer a setback. If that is the case, try to increase your laxative dose, use a glycerin suppository or even an enema. Sometimes it is best to go all the way back to Step 1 and start over if you can't seem to get your gut back on track. This may even mean stopping your favorite high-fiber cereal, oatmeal, and bread, if necessary. Or it may mean switching to a different type of fiber product for a while.

Remember that it's best to take your fiber supplements after meals and your medicines before meals or vice versa. Although the fiber supplement manufacturers recommend waiting at least two hours after you take your medicines before taking your fiber supplement, my patients say that this is almost impossible to do. More often than not, you will find that if you try to do this, you will wind up skipping your fiber. Also, food stays in your stomach for up to ten or even twelve hours after eating. So if you were a purist, you would have to take all of your medicines once in the morning, and your fiber ten or twelve hours later. Unfortunately, many medicines need to be taken twice a day; too much fiber all at once can also cause problems. Waiting two hours after your medicine is a compromise; because this is difficult to do, separating your fiber products from your medicines by a meal has worked well for my patients. However, if you have serious medical problems, you should try to follow the manufacturer's recommendations.

SAMPLE MENU FOR WEEK 1 OF STEP 3

DAY 1
MORNING:

2 cups Kellogg's Raisin Bran

EVENING:

1 rounded teaspoon of Konsyl

DAY 2

MORNING:

1 cup Kellogg's Mini-Wheats AND 1 rounded teaspoon of
sugar-free Metamucil

EVENING:

1 level measuring tablespoon of sugar-free Metamucil

DAY 3

MORNING:

1 cup Quick Quaker Oats AND 2 FiberChoice tablets

EVENING:

1 level measuring tablespoon of Fibersure

DAY 4

MORNING:

2 slices Fiber Five bread (Great Harvest Bread Co.)

EVENING:

1 level measuring tablespoon flaxseed

DAY 5

MORNING:

½ cup General Mills Fiber One

EVENING:

1 level measuring tablespoon of Hydrocil

DAY 6

MORNING:

1¼ cups Kashi GOLEAN

EVENING:

3 FiberChoice tablets

DAY 7

MORNING:

1 cup Nature's Path Optimum Power Breakfast

EVENING:

5 Benefiber caplets

The Role Age Can Play

For years, I enjoyed having people ask me my birth date. I would answer with a riddle by telling them that "a day after I was born, I had already seen two decades." Most people had no idea how in the world that was possible. After watching them squirm a bit, I would tell them that I was born on the last day of 1949 (December 31). So when I was one day old, I really had seen two decades. During my early years as a GI doctor, I noticed that I rarely saw anyone of my vintage in the office. Yet in 1989, when I turned forty, I suddenly began seeing numerous patients my age with cases of IBS, reflux, unexplained stomach pain, and the like. Yet I could seldom find anything seriously wrong with them. I eventually realized that the gut seems to undergo a major change at about this period in the human life cycle.

Although I am not sure of the physiological causes, I can imagine a few behavioral factors that may explain this change. At age forty, many people begin eating less to offset the tendency to gain weight in middle age. At the same time, the aches and pains associated with exercise become harder to ignore, leading to a less-intense exercise regime. But whether

Remember the movie *Pretty Woman*? Edward Lewis (Richard Gere) offered to rent an apartment for Vivian Ward (Julia Roberts), so that he would be able to visit when it was convenient. But Vivian wouldn't settle for that; she wanted marriage. Don't settle for less. We are talking commitment. Marry the fiber program. Follow the rules. This is the biggest mistake most everyone makes. It is true that you may do well for a while, but sooner or later unhappiness will most likely result if you only halfheartedly follow the advice given herein. The honeymoon affair with Benefiber and Citrucel lulls patients into thinking, *Hey this is easy. All I have to do is take some every day (or even a few times a week)*. I urge all my patients: Don't go partway with the program. Trouble is lurking around the corner if you do, and sooner than you realize.

it is due to these changes in what we do or the natural changes in a body beginning to age, around the time we find we need bifocals our bowel transit times tend to slow down. Constipation may or may not be more noticeable.

Generally, this is nothing to get alarmed about. If you are already at least partially on the fiber program, this new problem can usually be solved by increasing your daily fiber intake. Sometimes it is necessary to add a laxative such as a magnesium product or prune juice to give the shipping lanes a little extra kick. If you have never consumed enough fiber and are experiencing more severe problems, it is important now to take my recommendations to heart and get yourself on the fiber program. It is also a good idea to get checked out by your doctor

Get your mind around the fact that this is a lifestyle change, comparable to committing to daily exercise and healthy eating habits. All too often, my patients confess that they backslide because they were doing so well that they thought their GI problems had vanished. Unfortunately, sooner or later all of your problems will return, often with a vengeance. I tell my patients that with an excellent fiber program, they will feel like they have a twentysomething's colon. But real twentysomethings can do a lot of things that their older counterparts can't do, including getting by without a consistent good fiber plan. So typically what happens to many of my patients is that after a number of months or a year or so, they find that they can start cutting corners or even stop the fiber altogether and do just as they please. But this is not a good idea.

or other health care provider to be sure that nothing serious is going on.

From my perspective, there are two age groups. People under age thirty can generally get by on one healthy fiber exchange each day. If you have a bowel disorder, such as IBS, or significant constipation and gas, however, this will often not be enough. In this case, even folks younger than thirty likely still need a good dose of fiber twice daily. People age thirty or older should generally take a full fiber exchange twice daily (see Chapter 4 to understand the difference between a fiber *serving*, which is on the label, and a fiber *exchange*, which will allow you to switch from product to product without too much difficulty). These recommendations are generalities and may vary somewhat from person to person. Whatever your age, never forget that you are not taking fiber just to take fiber. You are taking it to get healthy results!

The following are my recommended daily fiber dosages separated into two age categories:

- **Age 15–29: one fiber exchange taken once each day.**
  Examples: 1½ cups bran flakes or shredded wheat; ½ cup All-Bran (Bran Buds) or Fiber One cereal; 1 heaping tablespoon of Benefiber once daily; or 3 FiberChoice chewable tablets daily.

- **Age 30 and older: one fiber exchange taken twice daily. It is best to divide up your fiber into roughly equal portions twice daily, about 8–12 hours apart. Examples: 1 level measuring tablespoon of sugar-free Metamucil twice daily, or 1 rounded teaspoon of Konsyl twice daily; 1½ cups bran flakes or shredded wheat for breakfast and 1 heaping tablespoon of Benefiber in the evening; or ½ cup All-Bran Extra Fiber or Fiber One cereal for breakfast and 1 level measuring tablespoon of flaxseed in the evening.**

Although this three-step program is the culmination of many years of trial and error, it should still be used only as a set of general guidelines. I am still learning the nuances from my patients. There is no exact formula. But many of my patients, even in their early twenties, are taking a full fiber exchange twice daily. These are usually young adults with IBS or some variation of this illness, especially with underlying constipation issues.

An Added Note

Be forewarned that excess gas and stomach cramps may occur during the first few months as your body adjusts to the program. Remember also that bad odor and excess gas means that your bathroom results are suboptimal, no matter what it looks like or how often you go. These are indicators that you may need to step up the laxative dose. Or if you have the dribbles (small little stools) all morning long, you may want to try a glycerin suppository or an enema, because the problem is that you just can't empty out like you should. Consider backing down on the fiber dose and perhaps pushing more with the laxative. Also, if you still can't solve the problem, try using a different fiber product, or going back to Step 1 of the fiber program, and consider discussing the situation with your doctor. If you have been on Citrucel for four to six months or longer and are getting to the end of the honeymoon period noticing increased gas or pain, consider switching to Benefiber (or EZ Fiber—more about that in Chapter 4) if you are having significant issues. Other suggestions to help with gas are found in Chapter 5. If you get a GI bug or can't eat for whatever reason, stop the fiber until you recover from the illness. Then get back on the program as soon as possible. However, it may be necessary to start back at the beginning with Step 1.

KEY POINTS TO REMEMBER

- **One hat fits just about everybody! A high-fiber diet means the same results in the bathroom whether you are an elderly woman or a construction worker.**

■ Forget what you have learned about whether a food or fiber product contains soluble or insoluble fiber. The fiber therapy program will help you select what works best to achieve healthy bowel habits.

■ Follow directions for the fiber program carefully. It was designed based on conversations with patients spanning more than a quarter of a century.

■ Start with Benefiber, Citrucel, or EZ Fiber. Synthetic fiber products such as these are less likely to cause gas, stom-ach cramps, and reflux than other products and high-fiber foods. But this benefit lasts only about six months for each.

■ Try not to switch from one fiber supplement to the next day to day or even week to week. Rather it is best to stay with your selected fiber supplement for four to six months, if possible.

■ How much quality fiber you are consuming before you start the fiber therapy program will determine at which week of Step 1 you should best start.

■ If you have been on a high-quality fiber product such as bran or Metamucil and need to go back to Step 1 and stop your bran or Metamucil entirely, use an intermediate dose of the fiber product and take it twice a day.

■ If you have problems with gas or cramps, consider stepping up your laxative dose or else going back to Step 1 and starting all over again. This may mean stopping your favor-ite high-fiber cereal or oatmeal. Also consider switching to a different synthetic fiber, but this would be the last resort.

Remember it is best to take your preferred fiber supplement after meals and your medicines before meals (or vice versa). If you have a serious medical illness, then waiting the recommended two hours as advised by the manufacturer should be considered.

THE MOST COMMON MISTAKES IN MANAGING CONSTIPATION

- Rushing into the fiber program too quickly. Remember, go slowly. Start with a small amount of fiber and gradually increase the fiber dose each week.

- Not taking the right kind of fiber twice daily and/or using an insufficient quantity of fiber.

- Taking too much fiber (see also Chapter 4 for the recommended amounts of fiber).

- Stopping laxatives too hastily (Milk of Magnesia, prunes or apples or their juices, MiraLax/GlycoLax).

- Waiting too long to start a laxative. Be proactive! If you know your bowels are going to slow down, don't wait to start a laxative or to increase the laxative dose. Remember, if you stay on top of your bowel movements, it will eventually take less and less effort to maintain healthy bowel habits.

- Not taking your laxative daily.

- Not taking enough laxative to do the job.

- Not using an enema or a glycerin suppository when nothing else is working.

CHAPTER 4

Filling Up on Fiber

Recently I had to buy a new laptop computer simply because I could not find a new battery for my old laptop! This is nonsense! Just as computer companies don't talk to each other, neither do the cereal and fiber product manufacturers. There is a fantastic array of high-fiber foods on the market, and if I were to try to list and analyze all of them, this book would be outdated before the first copy was printed. In the last chapter I introduced a tightly structured program to get you up on your bike, providing the training wheels in the way of the fiber products I feel will be most effective in helping you find your balance. Once you are rolling along pretty well, you can take the training wheels off and try your own fiber products. But how can you be certain that your fiber products will provide sufficient fiber to maintain the speed and balance you have achieved thus far?

In this chapter I level the playing field by introducing the concept of fiber exchanges. This way you can switch from one fiber source to another painlessly and know what you are getting into. For example, one cup of oatmeal is a serving, but its fiber content is not comparable to one-half cup of All-Bran, and the fiber content of two Metamucil capsules does not match that of the oatmeal or All-Bran either. I have read almost all of the labels and personally tried most of the products on the market (that I recommend) and will help you walk through this maze of confusing misinformation. My hope and expectation is that eventually the manufacturers and dietitians will get together and embrace this idea of fiber exchanges. If you find yourself running into trouble, consider going back to Step 1 of the program and starting all over again (and possibly rereading a chapter or two).

Mr. E exemplifies the typical patient who walks into my

A MIDDLE-AGED MAN WITH BOWEL CONTROL ISSUES

Mr. E was in his midsixties and came into my office for a colonoscopy to evaluate a rectal bleeding problem. He was in generally good health, and although I suspected that his bleeding was due to hemorrhoids, in view of his age I performed a colonoscopy. After finding nothing serious, I recommended that he try my high-fiber program so that he wouldn't be straining so much in the bathroom. A year later, Mr. E returned to my office and blurted out: "I've got problems! I can't control my bowels!" I asked how long this had been going on, and he explained that this had been a problem since even before his colonoscopy, but he had been just too embarrassed at the time to talk about it. However, it had gotten so bad he couldn't ignore it any longer. "Why, I can't even be an usher in church, because I never know when it's going to happen, and it smells so bad!" He denied any complaints such as numbness or weakness of his legs or significant back pain, and he did not have any problems with urinary control. This suggested to me that whatever was causing the problem was likely not due to any nerve damage, but was probably due to a functional disorder. A functional disorder is something that does not have a physical explanation, such as a spinal cord or pudendal nerve injury. As an aside, when there is a problem like this, rather than sending a patient out of town to Duke or UNC for specialized testing, I generally suggest a trial of the fiber therapy program because it is inexpensive and it also has a high chance for success. Those with poor bowel control who do not respond and have a poor response to the fiber therapy program are the ones I advise to undergo specialized testing.

So I decided to ask Mr. E why he was not following the fiber instructions that I had given him. "But I *am* following your high-fiber diet. I have great stools," he protested. His rectal bleeding had indeed disappeared. I responded by saying, "I know you haven't been following my program, because if you were, you wouldn't be having this problem." It turned out that Mr. E, like so many Americans, thought that fruits and vegetables were adequate for dietary fiber intake. He also mistook solid but foul smelling stools as being normal. As it stood, he had taken only a cursory glance at my recommendations a year ago and had not embraced the fiber therapy program as I had hoped. This time, after carefully adhering to the program recommendations, his problem promptly resolved.

office with preconceived ideas of what a high-fiber diet looks like and what constitutes normal bowel habits. I face this situation time and time again. The major reason why everybody at first wants to dabble with fiber and laxatives rather than to marry my fiber program is that they grew up passing small, foul-smelling stools and don't see this as the symptom of a deeper problem. This book represents a brave new world for most folks. Follow these instructions as if you are going out on your first bicycle ride. Sure, I realize that more than a few folks will fall off their bikes before they get the swing of it, but by and large, most will succeed if they follow my directions. The three-step fiber program is the closest thing yet I know of to a bicycle with training wheels. Once you understand firsthand what my program will do for you (and preferably for at least four to six months), then you can try tweaking the program to best meet your needs. Stay on my program for at least four months to understand what a good fiber program should do for you, and when you are getting those bathroom results (three to five large soft stools daily, with minimal odor), then you can try substituting your preferred cereal or fiber supplement. But if you want to get better, you need to follow instructions. Pure and simple.

A NURSE WITH KILLER HEMORRHOIDS

Eight years ago, a retired registered nurse came to see me for heartburn and "killer hemorrhoids." I don't think I've ever heard anyone describe their hemorrhoids that way, but I knew what she meant. She got the "fiber talk," and I really connected with her. Over the ensuing years, she has returned for periodic office visits concerning an unrelated health issue. Each time she returns to my office, she asks, "Don't you remember me? I am your Metamucil poster girl!" stressing how faithfully she has adhered to the fiber program. At any rate, her back had been to the wall, and she was willing to try anything that might help solve her "killer hemorrhoids" problem—anything short of surgery, that is. She has been well rewarded for her efforts.

There are three things about the retired nurse that you should note. First, she admitted she had a major problem. Second, she realized that I was the expert. And third, following my instructions wasn't so hard after all, and what the heck? Why not give it a swing? It's not like I told her to go jump in the lake or recommended surgery. Hemorrhoid surgery may not sound like major surgery, but it can be from the patient's point of view, as this is a very sensitive area.

Fiber Exchanges

Probably the single most important idea in this chapter is the concept of fiber exchanges. Grasping this idea is key for achieving excellent long-term success with the program. People with diabetes well know about fruit exchanges, vegetable exchanges, meat exchanges, dairy exchanges, and starch exchanges. Some people confuse the idea of an exchange and a serving size, but they are not the same thing. For one thing, a serving size of grapes varies in the eye of the beholder. You may think a few grapes are a serving; someone else may see a large cluster as a serving. But a grape exchange to a person with diabetes would be a half-cup of grapes, and not one grape more. Likewise, one apple would be a serving of fruit, but to a person with diabetes, half of a large Washington Red and a whole Rome apple may be interchangeable.

I am just such a stickler when it comes to fiber exchanges. A serving of sugar-free Metamucil is 1 rounded teaspoon, but as far as the gut is concerned, Metamucil's fiber content of

3.4 g of psyllium is *not* the same as a serving of Cheerios (1 cup, 3 g of fiber) or a serving of All-Bran (⅓ cup, 13 g of fiber). And for Konsyl, one serving is 1 rounded teaspoon, but it has 6 g of psyllium! In comparison, a tablespoon of sugar-free Metamucil contains the same amount of psyllium as a serving of Konsyl. Or look at bread: The serving size varies from one to two slices, and the fiber content of bread runs the gamut from 1 to 5 g per slice! So why not fiber exchanges? Thinking of fiber exchanges as outlined in this chapter will enable you to have clear sailing when you visit your local grocery store and whenever you are trying a different cereal or fiber product. As we saw in the last chapter, not all fiber behaves the same way in your GI tract.

Before getting down to the basics of what constitutes a fiber exchange, there is one complicating factor: Almost all fiber products have on their label not only the fiber content but the recommendation that you may take the fiber supplement as often as three times daily. Although this is all well and good, studies have shown that compliance with any prescription medication rapidly drops the more often it needs to be taken. For an antacid such as Tagamet that needed to be taken four times daily (as was recommended when it was first released thirty years ago), the manufacturers learned that few people could remember to do this on a consistent basis. It turns out that taking a medication three times daily is almost as difficult. Frankly, few people are willing to lead their lives around taking pills and watching the clock! Prescription medications that need to be taken only once or twice daily have the best likelihood of patient compliance. This means that if a doctor gives you a medication that needs to be taken three or four times daily to control your blood pressure, even though your life may depend on it, you will be hard pressed to take it more than twice daily. Likewise, dentists recommend that we floss our teeth twice daily, actually hoping that we will floss at least once a day.

So keeping this idea in mind, although I recommend the same amount of daily fiber as the manufacturers do, *I divide the total twenty-four-hour maximum recommended dose into halves rather than thirds* because for you to take fiber twice daily for the rest of your life is the best I can hope for. This means that my actual recommended dose of fiber will be 50 percent larger than what you see listed on the label of the individual product (the exception being Konsyl—discussed shortly). So because the maximum recommended dose for sugar-free Metamucil is 1 rounded teaspoon to be taken as often as three times daily, I suggest 1 level measuring *tablespoon* (if you use the big spoon from your silverware drawer rather than a measuring spoon, then this would be a slightly rounded tablespoon, but you should check to be sure as your spoon may be a different size) twice daily. The Benefiber label says to take two teaspoons as often as three times daily, and so I have changed this to be one heaping tablespoon twice daily.

The manufacturers of Konsyl have figured this all out. Whereas all the other psyllium products contain around 3.4 g and tell you to take it as often as three times daily, Konsyl says one serving is 6 g and to take this no more often than three times daily. So Konsyl's maximum twenty-four-hour psyllium dose would be 18 g; for Metamucil, it would be 10.2 g (3.4 g × 3 = 10.2 g). So the Konsyl manufacturers and I are on the same sheet of music. But I side with the manufacturer of Metamucil and believe that 10–12 g of psyllium per day is the correct amount of fiber. Eventually the other manufacturers will wake up to this immutable fact of human behavior and change their dose recommendation to 5 or 6 g of psyllium taken as often as twice daily. By the way, one Metamucil capsule contains 0.5 g of psyllium. So if you decided that you would just take Metamucil capsules to meet your fiber needs, this would be twenty a day. That is correct, twenty capsules daily of Metamucil is the same as 1 level tablespoon of sugar-free Metamucil powder twice daily. Yet the Metamucil container suggests that *six* capsules daily is the maximum daily dose. But if you do the math, this works out to only 3 g of psyllium daily as the maximum daily dose. There is a similar problem with Citrucel capsules; my recommended maximum daily dose for Citrucel would be six capsules twice daily (twelve daily), which equals 6 g of meth-ylcellulose, found in three scoops daily of Citrucel, the manu-facturer's maximum daily recommended dose. This is why I have developed this fiber exchange idea; hopefully one day the FDA will mandate a level playing ground for consumers, mak-ing it easier for everyone to compare products and prices more easily.

The labels of most fiber supplements also warn that they may cause choking if they are not taken with enough liquid. There are also reports that the back of your throat may become blocked, also almost always if the supplement is not taken with enough liquid. However, in twenty-five plus years of practice, I have never encountered this situation in any of my patients, nor do I recall seeing any reports of this in the journals that I read. So although this may occur, it must be rare. This same type of choking problem can also occur with the biphosphonates, med-icines that women take for osteoporosis, yet millions of women take these medicines in spite of this potential reaction. The key is to follow instructions carefully, and if you do, the chances of a serious problem such as a blockage of your esophagus are very low. You need to understand that fiber supplements such as Metamucil and Citrucel really work much like a sponge that has been ground up into a fine powder. These products are designed to bind water avidly (see Chapter 2). If you don't drink enough liquid with them or take too much at a time, then they may remain dry and thus may not move down your esophagus (swallowing tube) as they should. Fortunately, a cup of water or your preferred beverage should be adequate. Just use common sense! Drink extra liquids while taking your preferred fiber product (and, for that matter, with any medication).

Some people succeed on my program by taking all their fiber in one dose. They may take a heaping tablespoon of sugar-free Metamucil once daily or eat a full cup (or more) of All-Bran Extra Fiber each day. But these folks run the risk of getting into troubles with a fiber clog, because they take too much fiber all at once and don't drink enough liquid along with it. Also, because they are not sweeping out their system twice a day, as would happen with the twice-daily fiber program that I recommend, they run the risk of getting a gas lock, causing everything to shut down abruptly (see Chapter 5). From all those years of listening to my patients, I find that twice-daily fiber seems to work best—minimizing the risk of a fiber clog or a gas lock and optimizing your chances of consistently getting sufficient fiber in the diet.

Also, remember that although many fruits and vegetables are a good source of healthy fiber for the heart, they are not a good source of fiber for the GI tract, and in fact many "fiber" cereals and, shockingly, most whole-wheat or whole-grain breads have little fiber (see Chapter 2). For instance, two to three cups of oatmeal (depending on the brand), four cups of Cheerios, or three cups of Wheaties have about the same amount of fiber as one-third cup of All-Bran or Fiber One: 13 grams. And for that matter, few people (apart from teenage boys) can sit down and eat four cups of Cheerios or three cups of Wheaties for breakfast. So, even when you have good intentions of eating what you think to be a high-fiber cereal like Wheaties, you are still going to fall way short of the actual amount of fiber you actually need for breakfast. This is why you need this idea of fiber exchanges stamped clearly in your mind and why fiber supplements such as Metamucil or Benefiber could come in to help, particularly for the evening dose, if you have had All-Bran or Fiber One that morning. If you hate bran but don't mind Wheaties in the morning, take a rounded teaspoon of sugar-free Metamucil in addition to your cup of Wheaties. Or you could mix one-fourth cup of Fiber One in with a cup of Wheaties. In the evening, if you don't want to have good fiber cereal or don't like good-quality, high-fiber bread, I recommend one slightly rounded tablespoon of sugar-free Metamucil or a heaping tablespoon of Benefiber. (See later in this chapter for a chart listing the suggested fiber exchanges, in which fiber foods and supplements are combined into a fiber exchange.)

Another key logistical point is to leave your can of Metamucil, Benefiber, or your preferred fiber product sitting out on your kitchen countertop as a visual cue to remind you to take the stuff. Nine times out of ten, my patients tell me that if they put the can up in the cupboard, they forget about it and miss taking it as they should. But if you are nervous about leaving such a taboo item out, realize that it is a great icebreaker! Years back, my daughter used to be mortified that anyone might know that she took Metamucil, because she had had a rather severe case of IBS ever since she entered adolescence. But now she keeps a big can of the stuff sitting right out on her desk in her dorm room at Duke! Believe me, a can of Metamucil is a great conversation piece, and it allows Rosie to give her own version of the "fiber talk" to her friends and guests. I tell my patients in the office, "I am trying to change the world, but I can't do it by myself." So when you leave your Metamucil can out in the open, automatically there will be a lot of laughter at first, but then just maybe you will be able to help somebody in the process or nudge them along in learning about fiber.

Another way to introduce your own version of the "fiber talk" when you hear about someone's woes with reflux or gas is to say that you know of a doctor in Fayetteville, North Carolina, who thinks that everybody should "poop like a cow!" Once they stop laughing, you can add, "And he knows what he's talking about, and I can vouch for what he's saying." And then if you have enough bluster, you can tell your own story.

Yes, as odd as this sounds, we have got to get this bathroom talk out of the bathroom and into the kitchen. My wife, Lucy, tells the story that when she was only five, during a large family reunion, and at breakfast, her second cousin's husband asked his kids if they had had their "pancakes" yet, referencing bathroom stops. Lucy's mother was furious and later told Lucy and her sister to "never, ever" discuss such a subject in public, much less at breakfast! But I firmly disagree and would argue that getting this talk out in the open is important. As you will find from reading this book, our health depends on it. A woman told me that last spring, her whole family discussed my recommendations during their Easter lunch—perhaps to the dismay of some of the younger tykes! One of my neighbors who is a successful car dealer often manages at times to work in his own version of my "fiber talk" during business deals, and he feels it even helps him make a sale! People really want to know what they can do for their health and how to prevent illness.

One time I gave my "fiber talk" as we were returning from Machu Picchu on the train. My expanded version of the "fiber talk" was clocked (unbeknownst to me) by my oldest son at well over forty-five minutes—but hey, there wasn't too much else to talk about otherwise anyway on this four-hour train trip back to Cuzco. But if you don't want to explain your healthy bathroom rituals and don't feel ready to start giving out free medical advice, you can always buy a decorative container for your counter and transfer the contents of your Metamucil can.

Fiber Products and Good-Quality Dietary Fiber

Besides psyllium (Metamucil, Konsyl, and Hydrocil, to name a few), Citrucel (methylcellulose), and Benefiber (wheat dextrin), other good fiber products include EZ Fiber (guar gum) and FiberChoice and Fibersure (inulin). EZ Fiber is an especially welcome addition because it is similar to Citrucel and Bene-fiber, being a natural fiber product that has been chemically altered. For this reason, EZ Fiber likewise enjoys this same honeymoon effect, and indeed, EZ Fiber can also be used in Step 1 of the fiber program. It is harder to find EZ Fiber, but it can be found online.

Inulin (Fibersure and FiberChoice) is found in more than thirty thousand plants, so it is by definition as much a "natural product" as psyllium is. One manufacturer states that it is a "100% natural vegetable laxative extracted from the chicory root from Belgium by using water." Several of my patients (as well as my wife and I) have noted a problem with excess gas, which is why I don't routinely recommend inulin for the first step of the fiber program. But if all else fails, then I suggest starting with a small dose, such as one level teaspoon twice daily and gradually increasing the dose up to one slightly rounded tablespoon twice daily. Some folks do well with inu-lin, so I think that possibly the gas problem may be genetic or caused by some unrecognized environmental factor. Inulin is amazingly tasteless in just about anything, just like Benefiber. So it is a great product if the gas issue is not a problem for you (but remember that gas can present in different fashions, like reflux and unexplained stomach pain).

Other good sources of fiber are also commonly found in some whole-grain cereals and a few whole-grain or whole-wheat breads. The cereals are pretty straightforward. Read the labels to figure out which are good and which have only so-so fiber content. However, when you start poking your nose into the bread section, it is a whole different ball game. In the mid-1960s when I was in high school, there was a "brown bread" in the cafeteria that was always very dry and grainy. I remember that if I was really hungry, and if there was nothing else to eat, I would gnaw on a slice. At the time, I could not understand why anyone even bothered to put this type of bread on the table. Generally, unprocessed whole-wheat products such as bread and biscuits, if not eaten warm as they leave the oven, will very shortly taste grainy and dry as the remaining moisture is intensely bound by the insoluble fiber.

Most of the so-called whole-grain or whole-wheat breads on supermarket shelves today are big on advertising but small on substance. Be particularly suspicious of breads that say they are "nine grain" or "multigrain" and even "whole grain." This means they have a lot of different types of grains in the bread and even whole grain is also present, but more often than not the quality of their actual fiber content is borderline. For instance, most whole-grain and whole-wheat breads have only 1–2 g of fiber/slice, whereas others have 3 g and a few have 5 g of fiber/slice, which is what I used to look for when buying a loaf of bread.

But the problem is much worse. The grains used today for bread are not good quality, at least for my purposes. So even when you are eating a whole-grain, 100 percent whole-wheat bread or muffin, and even if the label tells you it has 5 g of fiber per slice, the fiber is still suspect in my book. This is equally true of high-fiber pastas. Why? No one wants to eat straw! Most of the "whole-wheat" and "whole-grain" breads are vastly different from those that were sold and eaten fifty years ago. Although it helps to look for grams of fiber per slice or per serving and not how many different types of grains of fiber a bread has, remember that the insoluble fiber content is not listed.

For example, Nature's Own sells a loaf called Double Wheat, which is listed as having 5 g of fiber per slice, but based on my personal use, I suspect it is closer to 3 g or less. The naturally occurring inulin (which is also the active ingredient in Fibersure and FiberChoice) has been added to this bread to beef up its fiber content. So continue reading labels and be inquisitive. But more important, notice what results you are getting in the bathroom with whatever product you are using. It just may be that whatever you are consuming is big on hype and not so big on quality. Please see also Chapter 3, which expands on this idea that the whole-grain breads and pastas that we eat today are not the same type of grain used only fifty years ago.

Remember, too, that if fiber has never been an important part of your life, chances are you are at least moderately constipated whether you realize it or not. Don't be a typical American and rush into fiber. Go slowly. Even if you are not having any GI problems, it is best to follow the simple three-step fiber program outlined in Chapter 3 and slowly work your way up to your daily fiber needs. This way you will be much less subject to gas and cramps as your body adapts.

Single-Serving Fiber Exchanges

This section is designed to show you what I consider a healthy fiber exchange for the various cereals, breads, and fiber supplements. Remember that my doses of fiber are based on the idea of fiber exchanges and your intake being twice daily, yet using the maximum twenty-four-hour dose recommended by the manufacturer. I have listed several different ways of obtaining a healthy serving of fiber and how fiber supplements can be used to complement your preferred fiber cereal or bread. If you are not on a good-quality fiber program, I suggest that you stop right here, go back to Chapter 3, and follow the directions for the three-step fiber program; otherwise you are quite likely to experience major gas and cramps. This is a process in which your gut has to learn to accept the fiber. Remember that it is best to start with training wheels before rushing off to ride a ten-speed bike. Once you are having excellent bathroom results, you should feel free to mix and match as you like according to your needs and habits:

ONE FIBER EXCHANGE:

BENEFIBER (5 g of wheat dextrin)

   1 heaping tablespoon

   5 chewable tablets

   5 caplets

CITRUCEL (3 g of methylcellulose)

Sugar free:	1 heaping tablespoon
With sugar:	3 level measuring tablespoons
Fiber Smoothie	1½ scoops
Fiber Shake	1½ scoops
6 capsules	

FIBERCHOICE (6 g of inulin) 3 chewable tablets

FIBERSURE (7 g of inulin) 1 slightly rounded tablespoon

HYDROCIL (5 g of psyllium)   1 level measuring tablespoon

KONSYL (6 g of psyllium) 1 rounded teaspoon

METAMUCIL (5–6 g of psyllium)

> Sugar free: **1 level measuring tablespoon**
>
> With sugar: **3 level measuring tablespoons**
>
> **3 Metamucil wafers**
>
> **10–12 Metamucil capsules**

FLAXSEED 1 level measuring

GNU BARS (12 g of fiber/bar; 8 g soluble fiber, 4 g insoluble fiber)

> **Banana Walnut, Cinnamon Raisin, Orange Cranberry**
>
> **Also sold at their website: www.gnufoods.com**

CEREALS (10–15 g of insoluble fiber)

> ⅓ to ½ cup **General Mills Fiber One**
>
> 1¼ cups **General Mills Fiber One Honey Clusters**
>
> 1 cup **Kashi Good Friends high-fiber cereal**
>
> 1¼ cups **Kashi GOLEAN**
>
> ⅓ to ½ cup **Kellogg's All-Bran Extra Fiber or Bran Buds**
>
> 2 cups **Kellogg's Raisin Bran**
>
> 1 cup **Nature's Path Optimum Power Breakfast**
>
> ½ cup **Post 100% Bran**
>
> 1½ cups **Post Raisin Bran**
>
> 4 biscuits **Post Shredded Wheat**
>
> 2 cups **Quaker Oats**

B R E A D S (10–15 g of fiber)

4 slices Nature's Own Double Fiber (See earlier in this chapter.
I suspect fiber content of good quality fiber in this product is
not as high as advertised.)

2 slices Fiber Five bread (Great Harvest Bread Co.)

The following are a few sample menu suggestions. Note
that if you choose one of the items off this list each morning
and evening, then you are getting adequate fiber for your GI
tract in your diet. Again, if you have GI issues, it is best to go
back to Chapter 3 and carefully follow the directions for the
three-step fiber program.

SAMPLE MENU SUGGESTIONS

DAY 1

MORNING:

1 cup Quaker Oats AND 2 rounded teaspoons of Benefiber

EVENING:

1 level measuring tablespoon of sugar-free Metamucil

DAY 2

MORNING:

1 cup Kellogg's Raisin Bran AND 1 rounded teaspoon of sugar-
free Metamucil

EVENING:

1 heaping tablespoon of Benefiber

DAY 3

MORNING:

3 FiberChoice chewable tablets

EVENING:

1 rounded teaspoon of Konsyl

DAY 4

MORNING:

½ cup All-Bran Extra Fiber

EVENING:

2 slices Fiber Five bread (Great Harvest Bread Co.)

DAY 5

MORNING:

2 slices Nature's Own Double Wheat bread AND 1 level
measuring tablespoon of sugar-free Citrucel

EVENING:

1 Gnu Bar

DAY 6

MORNING:

1 cup Kashi Good Friends cereal

EVENING:

3 Citrucel capsules AND 1 slice Fiber Five bread (Great Harvest
Bread Co.)

DAY 7

MORNING:

¼ cup Fiber One mixed with ¾ cup Post Raisin Bran

EVENING:

2 Metamucil wafers AND 3 Metamucil capsules

Remember, this is not an exact science. It is also best not
to rely heavily on bread for which the amount of insoluble
fiber is not stated, and most whole-grain breads do not use a

grain with high-quality fiber. Instead, I recommend that bread complement other fiber products and cereals. One other tidbit on bread selection: Beware that some labels list two slices as being one serving and others say that one slice is one serving— this is especially true of those diet whole-wheat breads, which seem to contain mostly air. Remember, we should be thinking fiber exchanges, not bread servings! There will be exceptions to this rule.

Fiber Five is one of these exceptions. Great Harvest Bread Co. says that its Fiber Five bread has 4 g of insoluble fiber and 1 g of soluble fiber per slice (based on a phone conversation). Based on personal experience and comments by my patients, I believe that this Fiber Five bread (also sold as High 5 Fiber bread by Great Harvest stores) is "the real deal." Two slices of this bread seem to work as well as any other single fiber exchange. Actually, this bread is one of my personal favorites, but one problem with it is that it tends to get very dry by the end of the week. Unless you have a large family (or one growing teenage boy) and can get through a loaf in a few days, you may want to freeze half of the loaf until you are ready to eat it.

I have also had little old ladies tell me that All-Bran and Fiber One are "dynamite" because they are getting fabulous bathroom results. And it's true. The problem is that people who are new to quality fiber products and foods who try to jump-start their gut with All-Bran or Fiber One can be in for a real surprise. I would not be surprised to one day see the manufacturers of All-Bran, Fiber One, and Kashi Good Friends cereals put up a warning sign—"Go slowly with these cereals, or they may cause stomach cramps and gas!" The All-Bran Bran Buds are a personal favorite for our family. When I travel, I take them with me in a small plastic bag with the measuring cup stowed inside the bag, and often I have them with yogurt or ice cream. The measuring cup is a nice trick because it is easy to take too much at one time. Remember that overdosing on fiber happens more commonly than people realize. Sometimes I mix the Bran Buds with Cheerios and often with Bran Flakes.

A *quick word about Benefiber, Fibersure, and EZ Fiber:* The powder forms of these products are just about tasteless in or on just about anything (Tea, coffee, water, mashed potatoes, and scrambled eggs are examples). A good number of patients have commented as to how surprised they were to find that they could not taste the product in their morning cup of coffee or tea. I personally prefer the taste of one rounded teaspoon of Konsyl mixed with one tablespoon of Country Time lemonade mixed with one cup of water. The other nice aspect about Konsyl is that there are no inactive ingredients; it is pure 100 percent psyllium. I like to say that Konsyl is Metamucil without the fluff!

Further Notes on the Fiber Program

If you decide to take one of these other psyllium supplements, remember that I believe that a healthy exchange should contain 5–6 g of psyllium—*not* the 3.5 g of psyllium that is recommended on the label. This amount of psyllium appears to be roughly equal to 10–15 g of insoluble fiber obtained from fiber-rich cereals.

Do not be afraid to be creative with your fiber intake. Mix and match the fiber exchanges in any way you like. The most important thing is to understand what a healthy fiber exchange is, but also to remember that you are taking the fiber to make those necessary bathroom stops for a healthy body. If you aren't getting these results, make an adjustment; add or increase the dose of a good-quality osmotic laxative, use a different fiber product, or even go back to Step 1. For most folks, the formerly mentioned fiber exchanges seem to work best. But it is also important to recognize that your body may require slightly more or even a little bit less fiber than I am recommending. Listen to your body. It often will tell you what it needs.

I also must note here that I believe that high-fiber cereals are the most effective source of fiber. This is not to say that you should only get your fiber from cereal. The cereals that are most effective include All-Bran, Fiber One, Good Friends high-fiber cereal, and Post 100% Bran; there are certainly others, but these are the ones with which I am most familiar.

Be forewarned that gas and cramps may occur during the first few months as your body adjusts to the program. If it is a problem, consider speaking with your doctor. Also, consider backing down on the fiber dose, pushing harder with the osmotic laxative, and even going back to Step 1 of the fiber program. If you have been on Citrucel for a long time and have gas problems, consider switching to Benefiber or EZ Fiber, and vice versa. Other suggestions to help gas are found in Chapter 5. Once again, follow the fiber program for the rest of your life. If you stop the fiber program for whatever reason, you should restart it as soon as possible and consider beginning once again with Step 1 if you have been off the program for a week or longer.

HOW A RETIRED BANKER FOUND THE GREATEST THING IN THE WORLD!

One day some years back, Mr. Y, a retired banker, came into my office to arrange a colonoscopy. He had just recently moved to Fayetteville with his wife, a former Hollywood movie star. He told me that he was eating ½ cup of All-Bran cereal in the morning and taking a slightly rounded tablespoon of sugar-free Metamucil each evening, and achieving excellent bathroom results just like I recommend to all my patients. I was surprised when he then told me he had been on this regimen for a number of years. I asked Mr. Y if by any chance a physician had recommended this program to him and if not, how had he figured it all out. He said, "I was out in California at the time when my brother-in-law from Fayetteville was visiting. He told me, 'You got to try this. It's the greatest thing in the world!' He's a patient of yours you know. So I did, and he was right about that. It *is* the greatest thing in the world." So if you don't take my word for it, listen to my patients. They are the ones who convinced me that I'm on the right track.

KEY POINTS TO REMEMBER

- Listen to your body. Sometimes it is best to start over with Step 1 and go more slowly.

- The fiber exchange section is a general guide. Don't be afraid to mix and match. The important thing is to get the fiber in *and* get results!

- High-fiber cereals appear to be the most effective form of fiber.

- Leave your Metamucil or Citrucel can out on the counter-
  top as a visual cue, and remember that it is a great
  icebreaker.

- EZ Fiber (which is difficult to find, but you can locate
  online) has a honeymoon effect similar to that of Benefiber
  and Citrucel.

CHAPTER 5

Banishing Gas, Functional Abdominal Pain, and Persistent Diarrhea

I n this chapter, the many different faces of constipation are unmasked. Once you learn to recognize constipation for what it is, then you have a handle on how to best take care of yourself. But also know that although constipation is the culprit, abdominal gas is one of its chief henchmen by which so much havoc is wreaked on our society. In fact, gas problems have been estimated to afflict up to 20 percent of our adult society, and I believe that even this figure greatly underestimates the extent of the problem, especially because you don't have to feel gassy to have gas problems, just as you don't have to feel constipated to be constipated. The surprise to many people is that they don't even realize that they have an issue with either gas or constipation. And if you don't know you have a problem, then you haven't a chance of managing it. The problems are compounded when one realizes that most doctors (including most stomach specialists) don't understand how to treat their

patients' gas problems and the fact that over-the-counter rem-
edies and medicines are more hype than help.

Managing gas problems is more than avoiding certain
foods or taking a medicine. What works and doesn't work
for gas and what foods to avoid and why are discussed in this
chapter. If you have stomach pain and all your lab results and
X-rays are negative, chances are good that gas is the problem.
Follow your health care provider's advice about getting yourself
checked out, but in the meantime, it may be a good idea to
follow the three-step fiber therapy program (see Chapter 3).
If an obstruction is ruled out, the fiber plan will most likely
help ease or even resolve your problems. If you have a noisy
stomach, frequent belching, reflux, irritable bowel syndrome
(IBS), explosive and/or persistent diarrhea, and even halitosis
(bad breath), chances are good that gas problems are at least
contributing to if not causing your problems. You came to the
right place for help. (See pages 108–109.)

So the rich are no different when it comes to intestinal
health. During my annual two-week visit to Bolivia, I see as
many patients with intestinal gas problems as I find back home
in Fayetteville during a similar two-week span. In my experi-
ence, intestinal gas problems affect all classes, ethnic groups,
and races equally. The exception to this rule would be groups
who subsist on unprocessed flour using good-quality grains.
This would include the Mormons, the Amish, and those in
developing countries who still subsist on unprocessed grain
and rice—either by choice or by economic necessity.

As the years have rolled by, my patients have driven me
to ponder the common problems of excess abdominal gas,

MY HUSBAND CAN'T HEAR THE
FOOTBALL GAME

One day, a socially prominent woman of Fayetteville, whom
we will call Mrs. H because she reminded me of Mrs. Thurston
Howell of the old TV show *Gilligan's Island*, came into my office
to see me. She had written on the patient information form that
her reason for the office visit was, "My husband can't hear the
football game!" Now most people write down things like reflux,
stomach pain, gas, or "My doctor told me to come"—but not Mrs.
H. She had her own style.

Mrs. H explained, "My stomach makes so much noise that
when we watch television Mr. H can't concentrate on the football
games. It's really embarrassing. I don't want to go out or do any-
thing, because it's just so noisy!" Mrs. H had regular bowel hab-
its, had no other GI complaints, and was in generally good health.
We scheduled a colonoscopy to check for more serious problems.

I next explained to Mrs. H that a noisy stomach suggested
intestinal gas. "Gas is a waste product," I said, and I paused for
a moment to let that concept sink in. Then I continued: "If gas
is a waste product, and if the gas is not moving through your
digestive tract as it should, then this suggests constipation to
me—even though you have regular bathroom stops. When your
leftovers move too slowly through your gut, bacteria can ferment
it and cause excessive gas production. So I think that your noisy
stomach is likely just a sign of constipation. Frequent belching,
bloating, and excess gas down below (flatulence) are other
common signs of a gas problem, and any of these complaints
also indicate constipation. If your leftovers are in and out of your

GI system in a matter of hours, the fermentation process occurs outside your body and in your septic system. You wouldn't think of eating rotting garbage, would you? That happens inside you if you don't keep things moving on through. Besides, if you can have a heart attack and not have chest pain, you can certainly have regular bowel habits and yet still have a constipation problem in my book." Mrs. H was riveted.

I advised her to begin with a small amount of Metamucil twice daily and to gradually increase the dose each week (Today I would have advised her to use either Benefiber or Citrucel, but this was more than ten years ago). I also told Mrs. H that her goal was to achieve several soft foot-long stools daily, and of course with minimal odor—much like what cows pass. If needed, she could take some Milk of Magnesia to get those results. As she had spent some time on a farm, Mrs. H was well aware of what I meant when I described what I wanted to see.

Soon Mrs. H's noisy stomach resolved. That Christmas, Mrs. H and her husband sent us a poinsettia that was so large we could hardly get it through our front doorway. They must have looked all over the state to find a poinsettia that enormous! Attached to the poinsettia was a handwritten thank-you note signed, "from Ferdinand and Bessie." I knew Bessie might be a reference to cows, but I had to ask my wife, Lucy, who Ferdinand was. "The bull" was her reply, referring to the classic children's story, Ferdinand the Bull. Mrs. H had apparently gotten her husband on the fiber program as well.

bloating, flatulence, frequent belching (aerophagia), halitosis, and rumbling stomachs (borborygmi). Gradually, the pieces of the puzzle have come together, in part based on my own clinical experience and in part drawn from published research on intestinal gas. At the bottom, however, is common sense. As this chapter will show, if one just takes a step back and thinks rationally about the problem, it's not all that complicated.

As in Mrs. H's situation, intestinal gas problems have many ways of announcing themselves.

Everyone should understand that your colon doesn't care what you think you should do in the bathroom. Your colon doesn't have a brain; it just knows what it needs to do: empty

AN UPCOMING TRIP TO EUROPE

Mr. W was an elderly man who came to my office with complaints of abdominal gas and distention. He was concerned about an upcoming trip to Europe. Mr. W's impaired hearing, combined with his preconceived notion of healthy bathroom habits, made my work more difficult than usual. Although he emphatically reported having excellent stools, from my perspective his bowel habits must not have been enough, because obviously putrefaction was creating a great deal of gas in his system. I fight this battle over what constitutes adequate bowel habits for my patients all the time. As it turned out, he was following my recommendations for fiber intake, but he was taking Milk of Magnesia only several times a week. Once he understood that he needed to take his Milk of Magnesia every day, he was home free. I understand he had a wonderful time in Europe. Most people with gas think that they have a serious problem, but most fortunately have just garden-variety constipation.

out all those leftovers before that putrefaction process sets in. You want to keep your GI tract happy? Then make sure you are making those necessary bathroom stops with output for which your gut is designed. Excess gas and offensive odor signify constipation, even if you think your bathroom stops are adequate.

Day after day, month after month, and year after year, I give some modified version of my "fiber talk." In fact, I have been told to put a billboard up on the All-American Expressway in Fayetteville, "Got gas? Go see Dr. Wes Jones." We should think of high-quality fiber such as Metamucil and bran as a vitamin for our GI tract. However, fiber clearly cannot be considered a vitamin in the strict definition of the word, a vital micronutrient that the body needs in order to survive. However, by using the term "vitamin F," I hope that the reader will understand how essential fiber and excellent bowel habits are to general good health and disease prevention.

So, if you have gotten this far in the book, you now understand that the most common reason for gas problems is delayed transit and expulsion of all the leftovers. With a well-tuned GI tract, undigested leftovers move on through and out in twenty-four hours. If not, then such leftovers sitting around too long can be fermented by hungry bacteria in your large bowel, causing all these gas problems.

When we are young, there is excellent gut motility and transfer of the undigested leftovers through our gut and on out of our system. This is largely due to youngsters' high food intake, increased fluids, and increased physical activity. However, as we age, the reverse happens. We decrease our caloric intake and fluid intake, the latter because our bladders are not as capacious as they once were. We also exercise less vigorously. All of this

A COLLEGE STUDENT WITH HALITOSIS (BAD BREATH)

Recently I saw Mr. A, a college student, in the office with rectal bleeding attributed to hemorrhoids. Reviewing his records, I also noted long-standing complaints of halitosis, GE reflux, and excess gas. His physician was perplexed as to what might be the problem and had sent him for a second opinion. All of his lab work was fine. I explained to Mr. A that he almost certainly didn't really have four different problems—bleeding hemorrhoids, halitosis, reflux, and excess gas. More likely, he had just one. I gave him my spiel. I also commented that Mr. A had a great GI tract. He came to the office thinking he was ill, when I was thinking that he was well. He just wasn't listening to his body! Sooner or later he would have to listen to it, and his long-term health would be much better as a result. It is the fifty- and sixty-year-olds that walk in for a screening colonoscopy with no GI complaints who have lousy GI tracts. They may listen to me and even wholeheartedly commit to my fiber program, but they will not get the same long-term benefits as Mr. A (see Chapter 10), who decided when he was twenty to embrace the fiber program for the rest of his life.

leads to longer transit times of those leftovers unless we keep our GI tract well tuned with sufficient dietary fiber intake and, if we don't increase our vigilance, promptly adding a good-quality laxative when necessary. If we don't, excess gas in its various forms is the result. How our bodies deal with this excess gas varies from person to person. That is what is so confusing to people and most doctors. But this is why as the U.S. population ages, increasingly more and more people have abdominal gas issues.

The question Mr. A then asked was, if this was so, why didn't everyone else have problems like his? I gave him the example of cigarette smokers. A few lucky people, on smoking their first cigarette, can't stop coughing or are overcome with nausea. They then refuse to try another. Others develop a severe case of bronchitis a few years into smoking, which persuades them to quit the habit. But still others continue smoking until they are in their fifties or sixties. One day, they have a heart attack, or perhaps they learn that they have advanced emphysema or even lung cancer.

Which of these individuals has the healthier constitution? The one who quit smoking after his first cigarette, or the one who smoked for years without problems? Some folks can tolerate cigarettes or a low-fiber diet for decades without problems, and others just can't. I submit that people who can't smoke or tolerate a low-fiber diet have the healthier constitution. It depends on your point of view. Fortunately for Mr. A, his GI tract was making all kinds of racket, and soon he would listen to what it was telling him. And he will likely live longer than his peers. On follow-up to the office, Mr. A was indeed better.

Although suboptimal bowel habits for our youth are not generally a widespread problem for the preceding reasons, a significant number of children have abdominal gas problems that often go undetected and untreated. Though I do not have extensive clinical experience with young children, anecdotal patient histories persuade me that recurrent abdominal pain syndrome (RAPS) and reflux are unrecognized manifestations of abdominal gas and constipation issues for our youth.

Until the early 1990s, I regularly saw children as young as age ten. However, as our group practice expanded, my partners asked that we restrict our practice to patients age eighteen and older, given their training background. Thus during my early years of GI practice, I found that if the child could follow a modified version of the fiber program, whatever his or her abdominal complaints, nine times out of ten the child did fabulously well without needing a lot of medicine and without having to miss a lot of school. The hard part back then was convincing kids that fiber would help their stomachs and to commit to the fiber program, and, if they were not getting satisfactory bathroom results, to add a quality laxative.

For some people, their gut can handle whatever excess gas is produced, and they may otherwise notice only a foul odor periodically. Other folks do not handle their gas nearly as well. When this happens, there can be bloating (abdominal distention) or frequent belching and even regurgitation of their food—what I believe contributes to or exacerbates gastroesophageal reflux disease (also known as GE reflux, acid reflux and GERD; more on this in Chapter 6). Still others have noisy stomachs (borborygmi) like Mrs. H, and many, like Mr. A, have a combination of these complaints. Research has shown that people with intestinal gas problems often do not make much more gas than other healthy adults; the problem seems to be that their gas just doesn't move through their gut as it should. This is why you may feel gassy inside, and yet your stomach does not appear distended. A little gas is trapped in one small location, causing the perception of a gas problem, but the X-rays just don't show much of a problem. On the other hand, if the problem goes on unchecked for decades, you may develop significant abdominal swelling. This is particularly true in the elderly, where we may occasionally find enormously enlarged colons on X-ray.

Many physicians hold that excess abdominal gas is due to air swallowing. However, to date, I have not encountered a single patient who said that by intentionally swallowing less air, his or her abdominal gas complaints vanished. On the other hand, when excellent bowel habits are achieved, generally the patient's abdominal gas complaints largely subside. So who should you believe: the physicians who tell you that your gas problems are your fault and due to air swallowing (which by and large will not help), or my patients who are convinced that the solution lies in an excellent bowel program?

Functional Abdominal Pain

Another major symptom of excess gas is, of course, abdominal pain. Just as heart attack pains can localize in your chest, neck, jaw, and even your arm, so the variable location and duration of gas pain should not come as a surprise. Sometimes the pain is on the left side; for others, the pain is in the upper abdomen or even to the right side. It just depends on where gas gets hung up in the GI tract. There are some medical terms for this type of problem: *splenic flexure syndrome* and *hepatic flexure syndrome*. These refer to the place in your colon where gas tends to get trapped. Remember that your GI tract is close to thirty feet long—but gas can get trapped almost anywhere, and this is why pain due to gas can be so confusing to people and doctors, even specialists.

Clues that your stomach pain is just due to gas is pain that changes locations (your gallbladder, appendix, and pancreas can't move, nor does an ulcer move around like that). Pain from appendicitis can move around some, but appendicitis rarely goes undetected for longer than one or two days. If your pain is brief, lasting less than a few minutes, it is probably a gas problem. Gallbladder and ulcer pain usually last at least 5–10 minutes and often longer. However, gas pains may persist for hours or even all day and sometimes even longer. Stomach pain that subsides when you lie down also suggests a gas problem, because gas can spread out much better when you are lying down than when you are sitting or standing up. On the other hand, gallbladder pain typically is worse when you lie down.

Fever, bloody diarrhea, weight loss, progressive worsening of your pain, and pain that wakes you up from sleep at night all suggest a more serious medical condition. But also remember that weight loss can be seen with constipation because the trapped gas worsens reflux and causes you to feel constantly full. Be cautious about taking any pain medication for a new stomach problem, especially if your pain is getting worse. Go see your health care provider and get yourself checked out. If your lab work and tests are fine, the odds are that you will feel much better on a proper fiber program, especially once excellent bathroom results are established. Start with Week 1, Step 1 of the fiber therapy program. However, in this situation (and only if you have been thoroughly checked out), to help mobilize the gas as soon as possible, I encourage my patients to start taking Milk of Magnesia or MiraLax immediately in addition to starting on the fiber therapy program.

Gas pains, especially on your right side, are often misdiagnosed as gallbladder disease whenever an ultrasound demonstrates gallstones. Having gallstones does not mean that your stomach pain is definitely due to a diseased gallbladder. I cannot emphasize this enough. Because gallstones are common, I don't order an ultrasound unless the patient history suggests a gallbladder problem and I am thinking that surgery may be indicated.

What causes gallbladder disease? Bile is produced 24/7 by your liver and secreted into your bile duct. There is a valve at the end of your bile duct called the ampulla of Vater. If you have not eaten and your stomach is empty, this valve is closed and forces your bile to back up into your gallbladder. Here the gallbladder concentrates and stores the bile. Storage of bile can cause gallstones to form, especially if your dietary fiber intake has been inadequate. Certain ethnic groups such as the Pima Indians (Native American Indians) are especially prone to gallstones and gallbladder attacks. So a family history of gallbladder problems suggests that your pain may be a gallbladder problem. There is also the "four Fs" tip that I learned in medical school: Being "fat, forty, female, and fertile" means that you are at high risk for gallbladder disease. Stasis also contributes to gallstones, so people who frequently diet have a higher risk of gallstones. The reason this occurs is because when people diet, they don't eat much food and food is what causes the gallbladder to contract and empty your bile out into your small intestines. If bile sits in your gallbladder too long, it can become too concentrated, causing a sludge to form, and this is how we think gallstones start.

What is not commonly known is that by their seventies,

men are as likely as women to have gallstones (15 percent). Another fact is that if you have gallstones, over the next ten to fifteen years you have only one chance in five of having a gallbladder attack.

Gallbladder disease can present itself in many different ways (just like heart attacks and gas problems). Sometimes your stones may get trapped in the neck of your gallbladder, or even in your bile duct (the duct that drains your liver and connects with your small intestine), and cause pain. Fortunately, stones trapped in your bile duct are relatively uncommon, but here they can be a more serious condition. So keep in mind that having your gallbladder removed does not always solve your gallstone problem. Unfortunately, because gallstones are so common, many women (and some men as well) are getting their gallbladders taken out unnecessarily when their complaints may actually be due to trapped abdominal gas.

Almost everybody gets better when their gallbladder is taken out, at least temporarily. Your gallbladder stores and concentrates the bile that your liver continuously manufactures, releasing it only when you eat a meal. However, if your gallbladder is removed, then your bile drains continuously into your GI tract 24/7. Then one of two things may happen. Your bile, unmixed with food, can back up into your stomach and your esophagus, causing what we call an "alkaline tide." This means you get acid reflux–like symptoms, and hence acid-reducing medications don't work as well because bile is causing your problem. Fortunately, this is not a common problem.

Bile can also travel in the other direction down your small intestine (when your gallbladder is out and bile does not mix with food as it should), ultimately causing mild gut irritation

A SURGEON WHO REFUSED TO OPERATE
ON A GALLBLADDER

Recently I saw a man with such severe stomach pain that he went to the emergency room. There his ultrasound showed gallbladder sludge, the sandlike material that is a precursor of gallstones. He was referred to a general surgeon, who rightly declined to perform surgery and advised seeing a gastroenterologist. The reason was that his stomach pain was not typical for a diseased gallbladder. It was brief, lasting less than a minute, and it changed locations. Given this history, it would be unusual for this to be gallbladder pain. I respect his surgeon for asking the right questions. Not all of them do. As it turned out, he embarked on the fiber therapy program and his pain did not return.

and, fortunately for the patient, better bathroom results. When this happens, gas symptoms often improve. This is why most people get better after gallbladder surgery (whether their gallbladder was the problem or not). However, gas pains will recur if the gallbladder was not the source of the pain in the first place. Of course, pain that returns after gallbladder surgery could also be a stone in the bile duct. So it is a good idea to see your doctor if your pain comes back after surgery. Sometimes when the gallbladder is taken out, people have diarrhea issues that persist for years. They are often told by their surgeon or medical doctor that the reason is their prior surgery. While this does occur, more often than not their diarrhea is actually once again constipation and it generally responds to increased fiber intake. Very seldom do I see a patient who convinces me that their diarrhea is due to their prior gallbladder surgery.

A WOMAN WITH UNEXPLAINED FEVER AND INTERNAL BLEEDING

Once I was asked to see a woman with internal bleeding. What caught my attention was that she had a temperature of 103°F. The story was that she had had a fever of unknown cause for more than a year. She had been to a major university medical center for a complete evaluation, but no diagnosis was made. The only finding was gallstones. I asked for a stat HIDA scan (a specialized gallbladder scan), which was positive. The gallbladder never visualized. She was rushed to surgery late that same evening, and a gangrenous gallbladder was removed. Her bleeding was incidental to the real problem, and notably, she never had any stomach pain. Her yearlong history of persistent unexplained fever also resolved. The point here is that you can have a very sick gallbladder and yet not have any stomach pain.

Look for a health care provider who will ask more than just a few questions. Don't get me wrong; a sick gallbladder can be serious business. Remember, your body doesn't read books. Doctors have to be detectives. Thirty years ago, before we had all these sophisticated tests to diagnose gallbladder disease and when gallbladder surgery was considered a major operation, far fewer people had their gallbladders taken out in a timely fashion. So we saw many more and very serious complications from gallbladder disease including pancreatitis, septicemia (bacteria in the bloodstream), and abscessed gallbladders. So if you have a gallbladder problem with typical symptoms, see your surgeon right away. Don't wait for complications to set in.

Today gallbladder surgery is very safe, with a low risk of serious complications. But if your symptoms aren't typical for gallbladder disease or if your doctor is not certain that the gallbladder is your problem, consider giving the fiber therapy program a whirl for two or three weeks. If your gallbladder is the culprit, your problem certainly won't get better on the fiber program. By then you should seriously consider surgery.

Why some people get one type of gas problem and others another remains a mystery. But this is the same situation with heart attacks. Heart attacks present in different fashions. One person gets arm pain; another has jaw pain; yet another has neck or even ear pain. One person goes to the emergency room with shortness of breath; another goes because her heart is racing; a third just collapses on the steps as he is walking into his house. Fortunately, physicians can recognize heart attacks much more readily with blood tests, EKGs, special nuclear medicine scans, and so on, all of which can document that a heart attack has occurred.

Diagnosis of intestinal gas problems is much more difficult. There are no laboratory tests to confirm a physician's diagnosis, and X-ray studies are only seldom positive. Also, abdominal cancer, ulcers, and gallbladder problems can masquerade as intestinal gas or functional bowel disorders. Intestinal gas problems, including functional bowel disorders, are what we call a *diagnosis of exclusion*. This means that other diseases such as cancer and gallbladder problems often need to be ruled out first before a diagnosis of an intestinal gas problem or a functional bowel problem is considered. Often I advise my patients that we will look for problems such as ulcers or gallbladder problems, but I suggest that they begin the fiber program because these tests more often than not are negative, and it takes weeks or even a few months before their gut has fully adapted to the fiber therapy plan. So why wait any longer than necessary to start the program? For many patients, however, a trial of the fiber program without lab tests seems appropriate, because intestinal gas and functional bowel problems are much more common than cancer or gallbladder problems.

Poorly Digested Complex Sugars

The second common reason for excessive gas is the inability of some patients to properly digest certain complex sugars. These complex sugars eventually make their way into the large intestine, where billions of hungry bacteria await a nice meal, with excess gas as a by-product. The three primary offending complex sugars that cause most of this mischief are lactose, fructose, and sorbitol. Don't worry. You won't need a major in biochemistry to understand what I am going to tell you next.

One of the most common of these complex sugars is *lactose*. This sugar is found primarily in milk products, but also in creamed soups and creamy salad dressings. As strange as it may seem, most of the world's population cannot digest lactose in adulthood. This is especially true if you are black, Native American, Southeast Asian, Hispanic, or Jewish. Cheese is well tolerated because it does not contain much lactose. Yogurt and lactose-reduced milk products are also much better tolerated than milk for the same reason. Most people don't realize that fat-free (skim) milk actually has a higher lactose load than whole milk. Soy milk is a good milk substitute with zero lactose, and the unflavored variety tastes almost like regular milk.

My wife and I both limit our dairy product ingestion to about ½ cup of milk each day. If we drink more than that, we tend to have problems with excess gas, and sometimes cramps and loose stools. It is truly remarkable how many people are aware of how common lactose intolerance is, and yet they just assume that they don't have this problem because they have been drinking milk all their life.

Most black people recognize lactose intolerance and warn their family members about it, but white people and Hispanics often don't. When my wife noticed that I was eating a smaller bowl of Raisin Bran for breakfast, she asked me about it. "I developed lactose intolerance a few months back," I told her. "I think I got it from that severe virus that Rosie [our daughter] had last year." "Do you think that may be causing all the gas and cramps I've been having these past several months?" Lucy asked. "Good chance!" was my reply. Of course, that was the first time that I even heard that Lucy was having any problems with her stomach. So cheer up; even being married to a GI doctor does not mean you will not have GI upset!

One remedy for lactose intolerance is to switch to soy milk rather than giving up milk altogether. For those of you who have never tried it, put aside your prejudices. Given what I've heard, I am a *supertaster*, a person with a highly discriminating palate. When I first tried soy milk, I mixed it with milk to disguise what I perceived as its unusual taste. Eventually, however, I acquired a liking for soy milk alone. Apart from its nutritional and digestive health advantages, soy milk keeps better than regular milk (at least until the carton is opened). One other tip, buy the unflavored soy milk (which tastes like regular milk). Most people don't buy vanilla-flavored milk to drink, so it puzzles me why most soy milk is sold with vanilla flavoring. It is, however, more expensive. Lactaid milk also works well for my patients.

Fructose is another complex sugar that is difficult for your GI tract to digest. High-fructose corn syrup is widely used as a sweetener for many beverages, including sodas, beer, and fruit drinks. Fructose is also found commonly in candy and other sweetened foods, but it is notably absent in diet beverages. It is amazing how many people I have seen over the years who had never made the connection between their consumption of carbonated beverages and their GI upset. One patient was drinking up to 2 liters every day of regular Coke and never considered that this was contributing to his excess gas and GI upset—not to mention all the extra calories he was getting.

Studies have shown that up to 25 percent of the U.S. population cannot digest the 25 g of fructose found in a 16-oz. bottle of a high-fructose beverage such as Pepsi or Coca-Cola. So if you have excess gas, cramps, or loose stools and you are drinking regular Coke or Pepsi every day (not diet sodas), there is a good chance that you have fructose intolerance and this is contributing to your problems. As an aside, sodas have been blamed for causing kidney stones and are hard on your teeth due to their high acidity. Drinking all of these sodas just isn't a good idea.

The third sugar that is poorly digested is *sorbitol*, which is in certain fruits including apples, peaches, pears, prunes, apricots, and plums. A way to remember which fruits are high in sorbitol is that all fruits that begin with an A or a P, except pineapple and pomegranates. All other fruits, such as grapes, bananas, oranges, and cantaloupe are fine. Unlike lactose and fructose, which may or may not cause gas or loose stools, fruits with sorbitol have laxative and gas effects for just about everybody—unless of course you are already on an excellent fiber program. Dried prunes are particularly effective as a laxative because the moisture has been reduced and the sorbitol is thereby more concentrated. Ounce per ounce, dried prunes are thus more potent as a laxative than prune juice. But remember that they do not have much good-quality fiber.

One day, a young, slender thirty-year-old man came to my office complaining of excess gas. When I asked what he was eating every day, he said, "I'm eating an apple a day." He seemed rather proud that he was eating what he thought to be a healthy diet. When I asked why he was eating his apples, he said, "To keep the doctor away!" We then discussed why apples and apple juice can cause excess gas, and why high-fiber supplements and high-fiber foods help reduce gas by accelerating bowel transit. So an apple a day does not keep the doctor away and may actually require a visit to one. As we shall see shortly, fruits such as apples, pears, and prunes and their juices at times can help your GI tract, but at other times they can be part of the problem.

For this reason, in the 1980s and until the mid-1990s, I was dead set against my patients using prunes and prune juice as a laxative; I would remind them that this fruit contributed to their gas problems (again, this was back in the dark ages when I was still trying to figure everything out and just didn't know better). I also discouraged my patients from eating apples, peaches, pears, plums, and apricots on a regular basis for the same reason. Subsequently I realized that if the sorbitol is in and out of your system quickly, then the gas from eating prunes may well not be an issue—this also is true for lactose and fructose. Also, some folks just obtained much better bathroom results with prunes and apples than they did with any other laxatives such as Milk of Magnesia and MiraLax.

One neighbor found that she got the best results for her severe constipation by drinking a quart of prune juice every day in addition to taking fiber, and excess gas just wasn't an issue for her. And a year later on the fiber program, she was drinking just a small glass of prune juice each day. This was pretty remarkable for a middle-aged woman who up until this time had only been moving her bowels at most a few times monthly, and this had been a lifelong pattern for her. So today I am much less dogmatic about my patients having prunes and apples or their juices. It really depends on what works for you. In fact, I prefer to eat half an apple (or sometimes a whole apple) or nuts (which are high in magnesium) to jump-start my system if I am traveling out of town or sleeping late on a weekend.

So it is important to understand that sometimes prunes and apples and their juices can cause diarrhea and gas problems, but they can also be useful for managing constipation. It really depends on your intestinal transit times. If you have slow transit times, then these fruits may cause excess gas and cramps. If you have excellent bowel habits and your bathroom results slow down a bit, then these fruits can help with the constipation and without much in the way of side effects. This is akin to the fact that a hot cup of coffee is great on a cold morning, but not your preferred beverage after working outside on a hot summer day.

Certain foods such as beans, onions, celery, carrots, raisins, bananas, and brussels sprouts have been thought to cause excess intestinal gas as well. For my patients, these foods have not generally been a problem, likely because the fiber therapy program enables patients to tolerate most gas-causing foods for the same reason as discussed earlier.

Medical Therapy for Intestinal Gas Problems

To date, all of the medications prescribed for intestinal gas are only marginally effective at best. One of the more popular remedies is simethicone (found in Mylanta Gas, Gas-X, and Phazyme, to name a few). What the manufacturers fail to say is that simethicone is an antisurfactant. This means it breaks up bubbles, but there is still the same amount of air in your gut after you take one of these products as there was before. We use simethicone all the time during a colonoscopy so that we have better visibility. Simethicone does *not* destroy gas or absorb excess gas. So as far as intestinal gas is concerned, simethicone is ineffective, and that is why most folks eventually figure this out and stop using it. I wish the FDA would intervene and set the matter straight. There is a lot of false advertising with these products.

At one time activated charcoal was recommended for intestinal gas problems, but studies are contradictory. Also, ingesting charcoal cannot be considered healthy for your gut, and none of my patients have found it very helpful. Beano contains a natural food enzyme that helps break down complex sugars and may be helpful for some patients. But seldom do patients tell me that Beano was a cure-all for them.

Finally, some researchers suggest that bacterial overgrowth of the small bowel contributes to abdominal gas problems and IBS as well. However, the research is not conclusive. Nor are antibiotics consistently effective for these disorders. Unless the GI tract is "swept out" regularly with a good fiber program, the bacterial overgrowth problem (if that is what it is) will continue to return. That is my position on the problem at any rate. In essence, I can't believe that periodically taking antibiotics for your GI tract will be a good long-term solution.

Probiotics (ingestion of live "good" bacteria) may offset this and other GI afflictions. Dannon yogurt is on the cutting edge of probiotics, from what I can gather. Probiotics are probably safer than antibiotics. However, since once again the underlying cause of the condition is not addressed, I expect that probiotics will all fail in the long run (see also Chapter 7). My thought is that if indeed bacterial overgrowth occurs in the small bowel, it is likely due to an incompetent or poorly functioning ileocecal valve (the sphincter muscle that is located at the end of the small intestine and relaxes to allow undigested food waste to move into your colon). Long-standing constipation probably leads to impaired motility of the entire bowel and thereby contributes to the conditions for intestinal bacterial overgrowth. If the constipation problem is never adequately addressed, my expectation is that whatever agent is used to solve the problem of bacterial overgrowth will ultimately fail. If you don't treat the underlying problem, you are just papering it over. That is my look at the crystal ball, at any rate.

Persistent Diarrhea

It may seem odd to include a discussion of diarrhea in a chapter on gas problems, but both are more often than not due to constipation. In my practice, 90 percent of my patients with persistent diarrhea get better with a good fiber program, and this means constipation in my book. Although I have some ideas, I am not totally certain why diarrhea is such a common sign of constipation, but I know that it occurs, and I hope these following case histories will help you accept what is a bona fide fact.

A BUSINESSMAN WITH DIARRHEA AND COLON SURGERY

Mr. B, a successful businessman, had had all but six inches of his entire colon removed only a few years earlier because of a high risk of colon cancer. Because the large intestine's primary function is water absorption, diarrhea was the predictable result of his surgery. A few months after his surgery, I advised Mr. B to resume his Metamucil (which he had been taking before surgery) but to take it just once daily. His diarrhea slowed to four to five stools each day, which was quite satisfactory, given that he was missing most of his large intestine. Then he developed a new problem—loss of bowel control and seepage. This was devastating for him.

The tip-off for me was that his stool and gas had a bad odor. So I explained to Mr. B that the gut regenerates itself after it has been injured, much like the kidney. Take out one kidney and the other one gets larger to compensate for the insult, enabling it to continue doing its job of ridding the body of waste products. So even though all but six inches of Mr. B's entire large intestine was surgically removed, he probably just needed to up his Metamucil to twice daily. Sure enough, by taking his Metamucil twice each day Mr. B solved his control problem—and as a second gift, his diarrhea and urgency improved further.

I call diarrhea that responds to the fiber program *functional diarrhea* or *spastic bowel diarrhea*. These two terms indicate that nothing is intrinsically wrong with the intestinal tract. Rather, this type of diarrhea is due to a GI tract that is not receiving an adequate intake of fiber and getting spastic as a result. Basically, if your diarrhea gets better with fiber, then

A YOUNG WOMAN WITH SHORT BOWEL SYNDROME AND DIARRHEA

Ms. E, a young woman in her late teens, was referred for a suspected liver disorder because she had a clotting problem (vitamin K deficiency). As it turned out, I discovered that she had a condition called *short bowel syndrome* causing this vitamin deficiency. As an infant, she had had emergency surgery with removal of a long section of her small bowel. At that time, the surgeon told her parents that her bowel surgery was so extensive, he doubted that she would ever reach adulthood.

As far back as she could remember, Ms. E had had diarrhea and episodic severe stomach pain. An X-ray examination of her intestines confirmed that she had only a few feet of small intestine remaining. But on looking at her X-ray films, I was struck by her small bowel, which was dilated (enlarged) with very thickened folds. Her intestines compensated in bulk for what they lacked in length. Her colon was also large—likely in response to the same surgical insult. Given her reports of excess gas and bad bathroom odor (a red flag), and even though Ms. E was missing most of her small intestine, I advised her to begin the fiber therapy program, and her pain markedly subsided as well as her complaints of excess gas and diarrhea.

it must be constipation. And if your diarrhea problem has been going on for some time, the probability that your diarrhea is actually constipation is about 90 percent. Hard to believe but true. Don't get me wrong; some folks are allergic to seafood or have problems with monosodium glutamate (MSG). Others have lactose intolerance, and still others consume too much fructose in their beer or sodas. But most folks I see in the office have diarrhea that is due to unrecognized constipation.

One elderly woman had such a brittle colon that it took me several years of cajoling her to fully embrace my fiber program before she got full control of her bowels. But now that she is living on the other side of the tracks, she is one of my strongest advocates. The gut is designed to live on an adequate amount of fiber, pure and simple.

Both of these patient histories give dramatic insight into how the gut truly needs an adequate daily supply of fiber for GI health. Like any other muscle in the body, the gut needs periodic stretching, but also powerful peristaltic contractile waves (contractions by the muscles within the intestinal wall) that move the leftovers through the GI tract and out of the body in order to prevent any gas buildup in the system. These contractile waves probably do not work as they should if there is nothing to push against, which happens when there is inadequate dietary fiber intake. The telltale sign of offensive odor and excess gas convinced me that the diarrhea of both patients would be helped with a good fiber program.

In two conversations with Dr. Martin Poleski, FACP, FRCP, in the department of gastroenterology at Duke University, he emphatically agreed that diarrhea can often be an unrecognized sign of constipation. I frequently suggest to my patients that the fiber program is a scientific test. If their diarrhea gets better, then no further studies are needed, other than a possible colonoscopy to exclude cancer and colitis. On the other hand, if their diarrhea gets worse, which happens with a small minority of folks that I see, then they are told to call our office for additional tests. This is a much more efficient way to limit unnecessary lab tests and to reduce health care costs.

I often hear my patients complaining of "explosive diarrhea," in which the leftovers typically splatter all over the toilet bowl as they spray out from the body. Excess gas is the culprit. Think of a rocket. It is propelled much the same way. Fuel combustion (food rotting inside you) generates rapidly expanding gas, which creates the thrust (explosive diarrhea). When you have just a few squirts at a time and go back and forth to the bathroom all day, this also is a sign of constipation. It is watery and you may have urgency, but not a whole lot comes out. Do an experiment. Don't flush the toilet, but wait for the water to clear and let the sediment settle. If there is not much fecal matter at the bottom of the toilet bowl, this is constipation. If you have food poisoning, perhaps two cups of waste material will pour out each time you go to the bathroom. This distinction between stuff just pouring out of you and exploding out is fairly helpful in differentiating spastic bowel or functional diarrhea from a colitis problem or an infection problem, in addition to bad odor and excess gas.

Another clue that your diarrhea is due to unrecognized constipation is if it comes and goes. Why would you have colitis some days and not the next? Colitis is an inflammatory condition of the bowel, sort of like rheumatoid arthritis, but it afflicts your colon. Colitis takes weeks, and often months or even longer, for medicines to get it under control. (See also Chapter 8.) Patients with colitis almost always have diarrhea every day. If you have colitis, you have colitis. It is there all the time. Your diarrhea should not come and go if you have colitis unless, of course, your colitis is under control with medication; in which case, functional diarrhea is likely also contributing to your diarrhea problem. Also, if you are not eating, then your diarrhea may resolve since there is nothing driving your intestinal tract.

With spastic bowel or functional diarrhea, you often rush to the bathroom but not a whole lot comes out. You don't feel like you got it all out, and often, just as soon as you step out of the bathroom you have to turn around and run right back in again. Other folks with this type of diarrhea just seem to take forever to get their job done.

I have explained how the difficulty of digesting complex sugars (including lactose, fructose, and sorhitol), could lead to gas problems. They can also lead to diarrhea. Some time back, I saw a young man in his twenties with Crohn's disease complaining of severe diarrhea extending well over ten years. It turned out that he was drinking at least 36 oz. daily of a carbonated high-fructose beverage (Pepsi), despite being treated by another area gastroenterologist. I told him that from my perspective, he might as well be drinking half a bottle of Milk of Magnesia every day and wondering why he had problems. Given that his Crohn's disease was under good control at his most recent colonoscopy, almost certainly his diarrhea was due to the fructose in his sodas and not Crohn's disease—but I also told him that some of his diarrhea was probably also caused by inadequate fiber intake. Sure enough, at his next follow-up

A PHYSICIAN WITH DIARRHEA

Dr. L, a physician, told me that he would spend hours in the bathroom with his severe diarrhea, passing ten to fifteen or even twenty watery stools each day. He also said it didn't smell and it was a large amount of stool. All of his lab tests and colonoscopy were negative. Dr. L was also following my fiber program carefully and getting an adequate amount of fiber in each day. The clue here was that it took forever for his bathroom results to occur—what we call "prolonged evacuation." He would spend thirty minutes and even longer in the bathroom just trying to pass a single stool. So Dr. L tried adding Milk of Magnesia in addition to taking his fiber, and his diarrhea and bathroom problems markedly improved.

office visit, those diarrhea problems, which had dominated his life for more than a decade, had vanished.

KEY POINTS TO REMEMBER

- You don't have to feel gassy to have gas problems, just as you don't have to feel constipated to be constipated.

- Noisy stomach, halitosis (bad breath), belching, excess gas, distention, gas pains, flatulence, and even diarrhea are often unrecognized signs of constipation.

- Excellent bowel habits allow the leftovers to move through the GI tract briskly, so the production of gas and foul odor is outside your body rather than within your gut.

- Lactose (in milk products), sorbitol (in apples, peaches, pears, prunes, plums, and apricots), and fructose (in beer and high-fructose sweetened beverages) are the second most common cause of excess intestinal gas and may also cause diarrhea.

- Lactose, fructose, and sorbitol-containing fruits have a laxative effect. These products can work for you (laxative effects) or against you (causing excess gas, cramps and even diarrhea). If you are having stomach upset issues, take a break from them and see how you do.

- Lactose intolerance in adults is much more common than generally recognized.

- Stomach pain that cannot be explained by your doctor is often a gas problem rather than anything more serious. Go ahead and have the necessary tests done, but also consider giving the fiber program a spin in the meantime.

- Don't rush into gallbladder surgery if your doctor is not certain that this is your problem. On the other hand, if after two or three weeks you are not any better on the fiber program and your surgeon thinks it might be your gallbladder, then surgery may be the best next step.

- Just because you have had major intestinal surgery and diarrhea, this does not mean that a quality fiber program is not for you. Clues are that less-than-pleasant bathroom odor and gas issues.

CHAPTER 6

Easing Heartburn and Asthma

A cid reflux and heartburn affect 15–20 percent of the U.S. adult population. Acid reflux (also known as gastroesophageal reflux, GE reflux and GERD) problems affect your quality of life as much as if you have diabetes. It's hard to believe but true. Moreover, acid reflux disorders can cause more than just heartburn, including frequent sore throats, hoarseness, sinus problems, and even a persistent cough. Reflux can also present as severe chest pain or unexplained nausea. Although medicines such as Prilosec and Nexium and surgery may be lifesavers, few realize that they just paper over the problem. You don't cure reflux with these medicines; rather, you control it, and sometimes even they don't work as well as you would like. Also, medicines such as Nexium and Prevacid are expensive, costing $4 for each capsule—ounce per ounce, they cost more than gold. Further, these medicines have the potential for side effects (more about that later on in this chapter), and most people really don't want to take any medicine regularly unless absolutely necessary.

Think of Prilosec and Nexium as being like the chiropractor who helps you with your back. If you don't do your exercises, lose weight, and do whatever else is necessary, more likely than not you will soon have to see the chiropractor once again. The same is true with acid reflux medicines. They are great for addressing the symptoms, but they don't address what is causing your reflux in the first place. So what's the solution? The fiber therapy program (Chapter 3) allows all of your leftovers to move out of your system, preventing the gas buildup that contributes to or even causes your reflux. This chapter helps you understand how to better manage your reflux, often with fewer medicines.

On one of my earlier trips to Bolivia, Dr. R, a Bolivian physician, had asked me to perform an endoscopy to evaluate his reflux problem. The test came up negative. At the time he was taking Prilosec for his reflux. I told Dr. R that that Prilosec was expensive Tylenol for his stomach. The Prilosec helped him feel better, but it did not get to the root of his problem. I next gave him my "fiber talk" and explained that many people have reflux because of excess gas backing up in their GI system, bringing all that stomach acid up with it. The solution was for him to get on a good fiber and bowel program and hopefully dispense with his antacids. Sure enough, Metamucil and *pan integral* (whole-wheat bread) worked great for his reflux, but Metamucil's expensive sticker price led him to look for a lower-cost alternative. Eventually Dr. R found that *afrecho* (chicken feed) worked just as well. On a subsequent trip, I learned that in

Bolivia there is also *afrechillo* ("smooth" chicken feed) for all the chicken feed connoisseurs out there.

Henrique Echegáray was the first Bolivian physician who bought into my fiber program. When we presented my "fiber talk" on a local broadcast, Henrique brought a large bag of chicken feed to the TV station, lifting it up for the benefit of the TV cameras, all the while giving his own modified version of my "fiber talk." My Bolivian GI counterpart in Montero, Dr. Victor Hugo Vásquez Lapaca, is now invited to speak about fiber and health all across South America, and he tells me that

AFRECHILLO! ("SMOOTH" CHICKEN FEED)

Señor V was a sixty-year-old Bolivian who traveled many hours by train for a return visit to my clinic in Montero. Every year I visit this city as a short-term medical missionary. On his arrival, he handed me a crumpled and heavily smudged sheet of paper. He reminded me that he had suffered from chest pains, had seen several doctors and undergone numerous studies, and all of the tests turned up normal. I had performed an endoscopic exam of his stomach (using a scope with a TV camera to examine the stomach and esophagus) on his last visit but had found nothing physically wrong with him. He was handing me my fiber program instructions, written in Spanish, on how to achieve better *el baño* (bathroom) habits. "I took that chicken feed for six months and everything did just great. But when I stopped it, my chest pain came back," he told me in Spanish. I asked Señor V to read out loud the last sentence on the paper. He read, "Follow these instructions for the rest of your life. If not, your problems will almost certainly return!" He then exclaimed, "You mean I traveled 2,400 kilometers just to be told to keep eating chicken feed?"

he currently recommends a commercially sold fiber product, Cofibran, which I understand is chicken feed designed for human consumption. "Too many of my patients were finding insects coming out of their containers of *afrechillo*," Dr. Vásquez explained. It seems that Cofibran is pretty much the same product as *afrechillo*, but without the insects. Indeed, fiber seems to be enjoying a greater resurgence of interest among GI physicians in South America than in the United States, largely due to the efforts of Dr. Vásquez, Dr. Echegáray, and me. So if you think you have it tough here in the United States taking your Metamucil and eating your bran, remember that you could be eating chicken feed instead!

What Is GE Reflux Anyway?

Gastroesophageal reflux (GE reflux, GERD or acid reflux) is a condition in which the gastric contents, including stomach acid, pepsin (a digestive enzyme), and recently eaten food back up out of your stomach into your esophagus. If your gallbladder is out or is not working as it should, this may also include bile, which has a bitter taste. A highly specialized muscle called the lower esophageal sphincter (LES) wraps around the esophagus at the point where it connects to the stomach. It works like a one-way valve designed to allow your food to move from your esophagus into your stomach and at the same time prevent your food and acid from backing up into your esophagus. With GE reflux that muscle isn't working as it should.

When the LES is working properly, it momentarily relaxes whenever you swallow, letting your food and beverage pass quickly into your stomach, and then it rapidly resumes its contracted state. Excess body weight (obesity) or pregnancy can contribute to reflux by exerting significant pressure on the outside walls of your stomach, in one sense squeezing your stomach and forcing your food and acid to back up into your esophagus.

Among the most common complaints from people with reflux is a burning sensation in the chest and/or neck. If the burning discomfort localizes in the chest or neck area, it is called heartburn. If the discomfort is more in the epigastric area (the midabdominal area directly above your umbilicus or belly button) it is then called indigestion or dyspepsia. Some people tell me that they have indigestion in their chest, but I record this complaint in my notes that the patient has heartburn. An acidic taste in the mouth and a burning tongue are other common complaints from people with reflux. Keep in mind, too, that sometimes burning chest discomfort or chest pain can be a sign of a heart problem, especially if your antacid does not provide prompt relief. Consider seeing your doctor as soon as possible if this is the case. There is not always a lot of time between when heart complaints begin and the onset of a heart attack.

Less well known is that reflux can also cause sore throats, frequent hoarseness, sinus problems, persistent cough, laryngitis, nausea, globus sensation (in which you feel like there is a lump in the back of your throat), dysphagia (difficulty swallowing), and even hiccups. One of our GI nurses in the office had been having intractable hiccups for several days and could not do anything about it. It just so happened that she walked by my office as she suddenly released a very audible hiccup. Up until then I was not aware of her problem. I suggested that she take a Prilosec with a glass of cold water, and her hiccups immediately vanished. Quickly drinking cold water through a straw is a neat trick to resolve hiccups that I learned from my son's third-grade teacher. But hiccups are also a sign of reflux and often respond to medicines such as Prilosec.

A number of my patients have told me that by getting their weight down even just ten to twenty pounds or so has helped their reflux tremendously. Studies have confirmed this observation. People also are often surprised to learn that breath mints (especially peppermint) and mint-flavored chewing gum often contribute to their reflux problems. Caffeine and a long list of medications also may contribute to reflux, by either impairing the stomach's ability to empty properly, impairing saliva production (which helps buffer any acid that may be in your esophagus), or causing the LES pressure to fall and thus not do its job as it should. For example, amitryptiline (Elavil) and others in its class impair the ability of your stomach to empty as it should and thereby may provoke GE reflux. Theophylline, an asthma medicine, also reduces LES pressure and so can cause reflux issues. Tobacco doubles acid production in your stomach and reduces LES pressure as well, so not surprisingly many smokers have more severe reflux problems. Other medicines have direct caustic effects to the esophagus, such as naproxen and ibuprofen (arthritis medicines), which, although they do not cause reflux problems directly, often cause similar symptoms.

Because the list of medicines contributing to GE reflux is quite long, rather than trying to list these medicines (which likely would be an incomplete list), I suggest that you discuss your medications with your pharmacist and/or your health care provider. You may even take the time to read the package insert, which will list all the possible known side effects of the medicine. I try to do this whenever I have a patient who has issues that may be related to a medicine. Remember that all medications have side effects, so you should weigh the intended benefits of your medicine against its possible side effects and then decide, with your doctor, what is best for you.

People often worry that a hiatal hernia may be causing their reflux. Hiatal hernias occur when part of your stomach slips into your chest, where it doesn't belong. Years ago, I looked at my grandmother's chest X-ray. She had a huge hiatal hernia, so much so that her entire stomach was in her chest. Yet she never had any complaints of heartburn or acid reflux problems. So although hiatal hernias contribute to acid reflux problems, hiatal hernias per se do not equal acid reflux problems. GI doctors talk about esophagitis (-*itis* means inflammation, as in *arthritis*, *bursitis*, and *appendicitis*). There is no such thing as "hiatal hernitis" because most hiatal hernias do not cause pain or discomfort.

Research has shown that hiatal hernias can contribute to reflux. But, short of surgery, there isn't a whole lot you can do about them. And surgery is still considered a last resort. Thus, the real concern should not be whether you have a hiatal hernia, but whether you have acid reflux problems. And it is better to work on reducing your intake of caffeine, sodas, chocolate, mints, fatty foods, alcohol, and tobacco, and on losing weight, plus following the fiber program.

Also, be cautious about those new endoscopic techniques for treating reflux problems. Somewhere in the world, at least four and probably more different types of endoscopic procedures are being used to treat reflux. These techniques are still considered experimental (by the most knowledge-able GI experts), and several of these procedures have fallen out of favor. Current endoscopic treatments for reflux include injecting glass beads into the wall of your esophagus, creat-ing an artificial LES effect; an endoscopic suturing procedure that works sort of like a sewing machine; and thermal devices that can "cook" the lining of your esophagus. These procedures have no long-term track record (few if any were on the market ten years ago), so although in the short run you may have some benefit (provided you don't have any serious complications), no one knows how your reflux will do ten to twenty years from now after an intervention like this. Because in all likelihood the endoscopic procedure for your reflux will be obsolete, why would you want to take that gamble? Also, if the underlying cause of your reflux (such as abdominal gas and constipation problems) is never addressed, I expect these procedural inter-ventions to fail in the long run and you will be back on your anti-reflux medicines such as Prilosec and Nexium.

Nissen fundoplication is a procedure done with a laparo-scope (that is, no large incision) in which your upper stomach is wrapped around your esophagus to create an artificial bar-rier to reflux. The Nissen surgery does have a long track record. Unfortunately, the people who do best with this surgery are the ones who also do well on medications such as Nexium and Prilosec. So if you cannot control your reflux with medi-cines, then your chances of a successful surgical outcome for reflux are also not as good. But even this surgery has its pitfalls. One study reported by the VA hospital systems indicated that 70 percent of veterans who had anti-reflux surgery were back on their anti-reflux medicines (Nexium, Prilosec, etc.) ten years after surgery. So surgery is not considered a cure-all for reflux, but it is our best gun that we have besides medicines.

This is where the fiber program steps in and changes everything. Because the program improves reflux, few of my patients request surgery; if they choose surgery, I expect that their long-term result will be better because they seem to have fewer symptoms of gas-bloat syndrome and thus less prone to relapse with their reflux problems. Gas-bloat syndrome occurs because after the surgery, patients can no longer belch to relieve their excess gas. Unfortunately, gas-bloat syndrome is common because the underlying problem of constipation, slow transit, and poor gut function was never addressed.

Smokers tolerate cigarettes for decades until they finally develop emphysema or bronchitis. Their doctor prescribes an inhaler to open the narrowed and constricted airways. As their lungs become progressively more damaged, over time they find this medication less and less effective. So it is with a lack of adequate amounts of insoluble fiber in the diet and a poor bowel program. For decades, there seems to be no problem. All is well. Then one day, heartburn arrives. Like the smoker who coughs but is in denial about the connection with smoking, the person with reflux is mostly aware of the acid and heartburn problem and not aware that it is due to an inadequate intake of good fiber and a suboptimal bowel program. He starts taking Nexium or Prilosec and does well, much like the smoker who uses his inhaler periodically. As the years pass, the problem only grows worse, and the medications tend to become less and less effective. Surgery may also relieve the reflux, but eventually reflux problems often return—all because no one ever addressed the fundamental underlying problem of gas and constipation. And if the reflux does not return, the person is still left with a gas-bloat problem, unless of course he or she makes a lifestyle adjustment as recommended here. Like the house with the water-damaged basement, the problem only gets worse if the fundamental problem of leaking water is never addressed.

Medicines such as Prilosec, Prevacid, and Nexium are among the most commonly prescribed drugs throughout the Western world. Some folks have many reflux-related complaints; others experience just one or two. GI doctors, myself included, have seen what seems to be an endless line of folks with reflux complaints, and yet there are few ways to confirm that their illness is indeed reflux, short of directly measuring the acid refluxing into your esophagus. Many people sound like they have severe acid reflux problems, but scopes and fancy tests rarely find a physical cause for their problems. Even if your GI doctor finds everything normal when you are examined for acid reflux, this does not mean that nothing is wrong with you. This is just one of those exasperating peculiarities of medicine.

Reflux problems are typically worse after meals, especially large meals with greasy foods and acidic foods such as tomato products and orange juice. Most sodas are also acidic, with a pH of 3 to 4. Reflux is also a common problem at night because lying flat allows your stomach contents to spill back up into the esophagus, like tipping over a cup of hot coffee, but this primarily occurs if your LES is not working as it should. One study showed that 70 percent of people with frequent reflux problems prefer to sleep on their right side. This is absolutely the worst sleeping position, given the position of your stomach in your abdomen. This is like turning the coffee cup upside down and shaking it dry!

Simply sleeping on your back or left side often significantly helps acid reflux problems. One of my dietitian patients told me that she puts a stiff hairbrush on her right side, which causes her to wake up if she rolls over during her sleep and thereby prevents her from sleeping on that side. A simple little trick, but effective.

Just as some people (and especially people with diabetes) can have a heart attack and not know it, you can have reflux and not know it. One man was admitted from the emergency room vomiting blood, requiring several transfusions to stabilize his blood pressure. His endoscopy exam showed a large, deep ulcer on his esophagus. From the looks of it, the ulcer had been there several months or longer. Yet he denied ever having any reflux complaints. Although researchers know a lot about reflux, they have overlooked what I consider the main issue underlying this disorder. For this reason, they are unable to answer the following questions: Why do reflux medications such as Prilosec (omeprazole) and Prevacid (lansoprazole) work well for years and then become less effective? Why do some people have more reflux at night and others more reflux during the day? Why do some patients with typical reflux not respond to these medicines? Years ago, it was said that Prilosec and Nexium are so potent in reducing stomach acid output that taking them is equivalent to having had major ulcer surgery. It is true. Back in the 1980s, general surgeons operated regularly for reflux and ulcer problems. Not anymore, and this is largely due to medications such as Prilosec and Nexium.

These are basic questions that need to be answered. I

believe that underlying reflux is constipation and trapped abdominal gas, which is of course due to a deficiency in "vitamin F." Let's just be logical for a minute. Why would your stomach contents move up into your throat when your GI system is designed to move food and acid in the other direction? Obviously, something is blocking your food from proceeding in the right direction, forcing it to go in the wrong one. When you are constipated, food stays in your GI tract longer than it should. This allows all those hungry bacteria to feast on your leftovers, thereby producing an excess of gas. Because you are more constipated than you realize, the gas often has nowhere to go but back up in your GI tract and eventually toward your throat, forcing open the door and being followed by all of your gastric contents.

All of this leads to frequent belching, reflux, or regurgitation. If it has a higher acid and liquid content we call it reflux, and if it is mostly air, we call it belching or aerophagia. And if it is mostly food, we call it regurgitation. In reality, they are the same thing. Belching includes acid and often small amounts of food; reflux includes acid, some air backing up, and often food as well. In the end it doesn't matter what you call it. If you get everything moving properly in the right direction, you will be amazed at how much better you feel. Furthermore, as constipation frequently worsens with age, it should come as no surprise that reflux becomes more and more severe as well. This explains why anti-reflux medicines such as Nexium often become less effective over time. On the other hand, once constipation and gas problems are under good control, many folks find that they can reduce their reliance on Nexium or Prilosec, and even do quite well off all of their medicines. This is especially true if you are younger and have a shorter duration of illness. Your LES is more likely to recover its normal functioning. However, people with more advanced reflux disorders and irreversible damage to their esophagus, such as strictures, Barrett's esophagus, and ulcers, will require anti-reflux medications indefinitely, especially if they have had reflux for decades, continue to smoke, or have major weight problems. Barrett's esophagus is considered a more advanced form of reflux where the actual lining of your esophagus has been replaced with a different cell type, which has been associated with an increased risk of esophageal cancer. For my patients with Barrett's esophagus, even if they no longer believe they need their anti-reflux medicines (e.g. Prilosec and Nexium), I advise my patients to indefinitely continue them, as these medicines are thought to reduce the likelihood of esophageal cancer.

The following is a note given to me by one of the GI nurses at the hospital where I work, which I believe says it all:

I worked as a GI recovery nurse when I first met Dr. Jones. Every time he came to discharge a patient and gave his "fiber talk," I would say to myself, "Oh boy, here he goes again with that crazy talk about fiber." I thought he was seriously a bit "out there," if you know what I mean. That was back in 1993. Meanwhile, I went through many years of suffering from reflux and constipation, because I was not smart enough to buy into the "fiber talk" that Dr. Jones prescribed. I took Prilosec and Nexium as often as twice a day (I tried them all), and yet I continued to have severe reflux. I often woke up at night coughing and choking, sometimes

*wheezing, and even having problems breathing. I used to
smoke, so I thought some of my problems might be due to
chronic bronchitis. I even saw a cardiologist and had a heart
catheterization (in which dye is injected into the arteries
of the heart to see if there is a blockage) because nothing
was helping my reflux. Both my heart study and endoscopy
exams were fine. It seemed that I was just going to have to
learn to live with my reflux problem.*

*Ten years later, I again began working in the GI lab and
I became reacquainted with that same Dr. Jones. This time
I worked in the procedure room rather than in recovery as
before, and I saw how he really cared. Not all doctors do,
you know. His sincerity impressed me, and this time I really
listened more carefully to what he had to say. His "fiber talk"
finally sank in, and now I wish I had listened ten years ago.
My life has changed dramatically. I no longer take Prilosec
or Nexium, and I no longer have any reflux symptoms or
wake up at night coughing and choking. I have regular
bowel habits and feel so much better now that I finally
decided to smarten up and listen to the doctor whom I had
once thought to be a "crazy man." I thank God for granting
me the wisdom to listen to what Dr. Jones had to say and for
allowing me to act on it. I feel like a new person.*

*Denise Carpenter, RN, former GI lab charge nurse
Highsmith-Rainey Memorial Hospital
Cape Fear Valley Health System*

I have not actually seen Ms. Carpenter as a patient, but I
suppose I have been treating her medical problems by proxy.

Today's researchers have consistently overlooked the connection between a low-fiber diet, poor bowel habits, and abdominal gas and reflux. Thirty-five years ago, Dr. Denis Burkitt concluded that based on his own research, GE reflux, hiatal hernias, low-fiber diets, delayed intestinal transit of leftovers, and suboptimal bowel habits were intrinsically related. The missing link for Dr. Burkitt was the development of a fiber program that allows people to adapt to a high-fiber diet as painlessly as possible. So convinced was Dr. Burkitt that physicians were headed in the wrong direction that one of his favorite cartoons that he presented at medical conferences was that of two physicians busily mopping the floor from an overflowing sink, but they never bother to turn off the faucet or work on the blocked drain! He compared this behavior of physicians to doing surgery for reflux or prescribing medications. Fixing the blocked drain (constipation and gas) would do more to help people than all the medicines and surgeries (mopping up the floor) combined. I agree completely with Dr. Burkitt's analogy. Although the specific example here is reflux, as this book shows, people with reflux are only one demographic that could benefit from the fiber therapy program.

So why do some people experience reflux at night, and others during the day? Reflux at night makes sense if your LES is not working as it should. All your trapped air is spreading out when you lie down, so for those with reflux issues, the gas backs up into the esophagus. But for those who have reflux during the daytime, my explanation would be that their gas is creating an airlock in the GI tract, forcing some of the gas to back up in the system. Also, they frequently belch in an attempt to relieve the trapped air, whether they consciously realize what they are doing or not. Several patients have told me that they had not realized how much belching they were doing until I asked about it in the office.

When I left Duke in 1983, we had a list of recommendations for people with reflux. First, for nighttime reflux patients we suggested elevating the head of the bed 6–8 inches. I soon heard back that their mattresses were more often than not on the floor, and they also tended to slide off the wedge intended to keep their bodies at such an incline! So I suggested trying 4–6 inches. Again, the same complaints. Eventually for them, elevating the head of their bed 2–4 inches was most workable, at least long-term. At this level, there were fewer complaints of leg swelling, mattress migration, and such. If you use an extra pillow or two, you will likely be sleeping flat by the time you wake up in the morning. Also, sleeping with extra pillows puts a lot of stress on your neck. The mattress wedge works pretty well, but I worry that the wedge may be tougher on your back.

You should also wait at least several hours after eating before going to bed and avoid tight-fitting garments and large meals in the evening. And whether you have nighttime or daytime reflux, avoid orange-flavored Metamucil and Citrucel products. I will never forget the skeptical reply by one retired Methodist minister who said that he had been taking orange-flavored Metamucil for more than twenty years, and it had never given him any problems. So he could not believe that this was the problem. I told him to just humor me and try using unflavored Metamucil or take Konsyl. And sure enough, his acid reflux resolved. On his next visit to the office, he shook his head in surprise that this tiny change made such a difference.

Ditto for chewing mint-flavored gum, drinking sodas regularly, and smoking.

Alcohol (if taken regularly and even in modest amounts) and tobacco are also terrible on the stomach. So limit your alcohol use and of course stop smoking. Alcohol is a disinfectant. Alcohol is what is used to wipe your arm just before your blood is drawn for lab work. Because it's a disinfectant, it kills all the bacteria on your arm so that the blood can be safely drawn without risk of an infection. Alcohol also acts as a diuretic, a "fluid pill." In college we had a saying: You don't buy beer, you rent it. Because alcohol is not effectively broken down by your stomach acid, it is killing the cells lining your esophagus and stomach and, not surprisingly, exacerbating your reflux problems. Alcohol can also cause your LES not to work properly. People are often surprised when I suggest that their reflux and heartburn may be due to the nightcap or glass of wine they have each evening. I remind them that they can't do what they could twenty years ago, and just because they could drink several glasses of wine or beer without problems back then, this does not mean they can do it today.

This is particularly true if you take prescription or over-the-counter medicines on a daily basis. We call them pills, but they are chemicals, especially arthritis medicines such as ibuprofen and naproxen. Lithium, quinidine, and certain antibiotics such as Septra, Bactrim, and doxycycline are also quite tough on your stomach. Even a plain old multivitamin containing minerals may cause a problem. One young woman in her late twenties, an employee of an area physician's office, was referred for an esophageal mass noted on her chest CT scan. A day earlier, she had awakened in the morning with severe chest pain, especially when she swallowed. When I looked inside her with a scope, I found a swollen area in the middle of her esophagus with a hole the size of a pill. It turned out that she had swallowed an 800-mg Motrin tablet the night before and then gone straight to bed. I suspect that it just sat in her esophagus all night long and eventually burned its way through. She could have died from this serious injury. I saw another young, trim woman in the hospital for severe anemia and difficulty swallowing. She had a lifelong severe back problem that years earlier had required surgical placement of steel rods. She had taken arthritis medicines for years, and eventually she developed a severe swallowing problem, a stricture of her esophagus. An endoscopy showed that her esophagus was so tight that it was about the diameter of the lead core of a pencil. No wonder she couldn't eat regular food like everyone else! She has required numerous dilations (stretches) of her esophagus to get her swallowing back toward normal.

People need to respect their medicines, even over-the-counter remedies. Perhaps fifteen years back, another woman had an ulcer on her esophagus that I thought was caused by her lithium. She said her psychiatrist had reviewed the world's literature and had run across only three other patients who had a similar problem—he had never heard of this before. She asked me how I had figured out that the lithium was her problem. I then told her about my science class when I was in the tenth grade, back in the mid-1960s. Our teacher had everyone stand back, and then she dropped a small piece of lithium into a big tub of water. Fire spurted out when the lithium hit the water because of a chemical reaction. Now I am sure that the manufacturer of lithium prepares it the best way possible to protect patients from this type of reaction. Yet most patients pop their lithium tablets without giving it a second thought.

I had another young woman who was taking the antibiotic doxycycline for her acne. One day she suddenly began having problems with painful swallowing. Endoscopy revealed two large ulcers on her esophagus, which I am certain were caused by the doxycycline, because this has been reported to occur with this medication. A number of other medicines can do this, and it would be nearly impossible to remember them all. So the best thing to do is always to remember to take your pills standing or sitting up with several extra swallows of liquid to be certain they pass on through your esophagus. Don't just pop a pill and go right to bed, assuming that everything will be okay in the morning. A healthy respect for whatever medicine you are taking is just common sense.

And remember also that alcohol and tobacco enhance the abilities of your medicines to cause ulcers, especially as you age. This means that if you take an arthritis medicine every day, which may cause ulcers, you are more likely to develop an ulcer if you are smoking or drinking alcohol as well—even if you have your alcohol at a different time of day from your medicines.

Fiber, Reflux, and Asthma

Medical experts have estimated that about half of people with asthma also have reflux problems. In fact, the more severe your asthma, the more likely reflux may be contributing to your illness. Of further note, many people with asthma are not aware that they even have reflux. Also, it is now generally

A TRANSLATOR WHO TOOK METAMUCIL FOR ASTHMA

Ms. E, a forty-year-old translator living in the foothills of the Smoky Mountains, traveled regularly with us on our mission trips to Bolivia. One spring, Ms. E e-mailed me that she could not join our group that summer because her asthma had become difficult to manage. Although I was not her regular doctor, I suspected that she might have a reflux problem. At any rate, I e-mailed Ms. E and asked her if she was on my fiber program. Of note, she had given my fiber and reflux spiel in Spanish hundreds of times while in Bolivia on prior trips. However, I doubted that Ms. E was aware that reflux could worsen or even cause asthma. It turned out that Ms. E had not taken my fiber program to heart. In the end, her asthma turned out to be just the catalyst she needed to commit herself to the fiber program. And sure enough, her asthma got much better, enabling her to join us for the trip that summer. While in Bolivia, Ms. E walked up to me one day with a big grin on her face and proudly announced that when she last saw her doctor, he had asked if she was using her inhalers for her asthma. To this question, she enthusiastically reported, "No! I take Metamucil!" Strange as it may seem, constipation and a poor bowel program may indeed contribute to asthma problems.

recommended that people with severe asthma be evaluated for reflux and aggressively treated if it is found. But the experts also acknowledge that people with asthma may have no complaints that suggest reflux is even an issue. However, if you have reflux, treating your reflux may not help your asthma.

Why would reflux worsen your asthma? First, the bottom of your throat splits into two tubes: One goes into your esophagus and connects to your stomach, and the other becomes your trachea or windpipe and travels out into your lungs. When you have reflux, the acid and foodstuffs in your stomach can make their way all the way up to the back of your throat. Here they can cause sore throat, burning tongue, and even dental and sinus problems. Some of the acid and food material may also slide into your windpipe and irritate your vocal cords, causing wheezing and even stridor (a harsh sound caused by a partial airway obstruction), and even possibly get into your lungs.

Although people with asthma may not have any reflux complaints, sometimes there are clues pointing to its presence. These clues include asthma symptoms that are worse at night, especially just after going to bed (remember that reflux is often worse when you are recumbent and especially if you sleep on your right side), frequent hoarseness, recurrent sore throats,

A NURSE WITH STRIDOR

One morning I walked into room three of the GI lab at Highsmith-Rainey Memorial Hospital, where I heard the unmistakable sound of stridor as one of the GI nurses was trying to inhale. She thought this was caused by her smoking problem, when in reality she had a severe reflux problem that was causing her vocal cords to go into spasm. I urged her to start taking Nexium twice daily and to embrace the fiber program (in addition to stopping the tobacco!). Getting off the cigarettes was difficult, but her stridor is no longer an issue. She will also now tell you that her reflux always does so much better as long as she doesn't get slack about the fiber program. She also does not need her reflux medicines as she did at first. Subsequently her whole family has been in to see me, so convinced is she of the benefits of the fiber therapy program.

A YOUNG WOMAN WITH SEVERE ASTHMA AND SEVERE REFLUX

Another young woman appeared to be almost drowning in her reflux. She had severe asthma and was on six or eight medications, including prednisone. She was making almost weekly trips to the emergency room, resulting in multiple hospital stays. Finally, someone sent her to be checked out for reflux. Once she got on a good anti-reflux and fiber therapy program, her asthma came under control. Of course, she was also put on Prilosec. Soon she was able to cut her asthma medications in half. She also stopped making all those frequent trips to the emergency room. I can't fully explain all the connections between asthma and reflux, but the idea to come away with here is that for one out of two people with asthma, reflux may be contributing to at least a portion of their illness. And don't forget that reflux is often caused by inadequate dietary fiber intake and suboptimal bathroom habits.

sinus problems, and a lump in the throat. Also, asthma that is provoked by eating a large meal late at night suggests that reflux may be behind your illness.

WARNING SIGNS FOR GE REFLUX

- Difficult swallowing, especially if this is a new complaint or getting worse
- Painful swallowing
- Weight loss
- Black stools (like tar) or anemia
- Heartburn or reflux that is not responding to treatment

KEY POINTS TO REMEMBER

- Reflux is often caused by or worsened by constipation and excess gas, whether or not you think you have a problem in that department.

- A good fiber program can help improve your reflux and heartburn, and may even allow you to stop your medicines for reflux entirely. However, sometimes during the first few weeks of the fiber program, your reflux may get worse before it gets better. You may need your reflux medicines twice daily as your GI tract adapts to the fiber program.

- Caffeine, mints and mint-flavored gum, chocolate, coffee, tea, acidic foods, fatty foods, tobacco, carbonated sodas, and alcohol may provoke reflux.

- Don't sleep on your right side, wait several hours after eating before going to bed, and put the head of your bed up several inches.

- Weight loss and not wearing tight fitting clothes also can help your reflux.

- Take extra swallows of liquids with *all* medications.

- About half of people with asthma have reflux, and controlling reflux may help their asthma.

- The more severe your asthma, the more likely reflux is contributing to your asthma.

CHAPTER 7

Relieving Irritable Bowel Syndrome (IBS)

When I was in medical school, I was taught that every specialty has at least one common illness that no one can fix. For gastroenterology, it is irritable bowel syndrome (IBS). For orthopedics, it is low back pain. For neurology, it is headaches; for cardiology, it is noncardiac chest pain; and so forth. This means that whatever specialty you choose, you will have an office filled with patients whom you won't really be able to help. There is nothing more difficult for a physician than feeling powerless as you listen to your patients' complaints that point to an issue for which little help exists. Many years back, I had one such day with an office full of patients where no one seemed to be getting better, no matter what their problem was. Toward the end of that day, one of my patients asked me how I was doing. I thought for a moment and commented that I was doing pretty well when the day started, but now I was beginning to wonder.

IBS affects members of both sexes and all age groups and is

found everywhere in the world. IBS comprises about 10–15 percent of the U.S. adult population, and one study estimated that the figure was even higher at 20 percent. In the United States, younger patients and women are more likely to be diagnosed with IBS, and there is roughly a 2:1 female-to-male predominance. Between 25 and 40 percent of the referrals to a gastroenterologist are for an IBS-related problem. Because IBS is a disorder that is widely believed not to have a cure, the goal has become to help patients learn how to cope with their illness.

Thirty years after I finished med school, IBS continues to be the bane of gastroenterology. However, unlike my peers, I actually enjoy seeing patients with IBS because I have found the illness generally very treatable, and most of my patients are very motivated once they understand that they have found help.

Imagine a woman who has had IBS for years who comes into my office for an initial evaluation. I am only the most recent in a long line of doctors she has consulted, and perhaps she is only partway listening to what I am telling her. "You've got to forget whatever you thought you knew about your body!" I say, keeping an eye on how close she is listening. There comes a certain point during the conversation, however, when I notice that a light has come into her eyes. Then I know that she has realized that there just may be help for her problem.

What Is IBS?

IBS is an intestinal disorder with periodic or persistent bouts of abdominal pain. It is always associated with altered bathroom habits in the absence of any known physical illness. If for the preceding several months (or longer), you have noticed a change in your bowel habits toward more frequent stools, smaller stools, diarrhea, or even constipation AND if you also have stomach pain, you most likely have IBS, provided your health care provider rules out other conditions. Stomach pain and an alteration in your bowel habits is required for the diagnosis to be made. If you have periodic episodes of diarrhea or significant problems with constipation, but no stomach pain issues, you don't have IBS. Also, if you have stomach pain and no changes in your bowel habits, you don't have IBS. Patients with IBS also do not show any significant findings on either a colonoscopy or a CT scan, or in any other lab studies for that matter.

So, unfortunately, there are no lab tests, ultrasounds, CT scans, or colonoscopies that will help your doctor diagnose IBS. In fact, the older you are, the more concerned your doctor will become that something more serious may be going on. Perhaps you have more pronounced gas issues or rectal bleeding, and your GI specialist has to rethink your diagnosis so as to rule out cancer, stomach ulcers, or gallbladder disease. If you feel like your GI doctor just keeps running tests on you all the time, now you know why. It is like a tension headache. Everybody knows people can get tension headaches, but you sure can't prove it by looking at the brain with a CT scan or under a microscope. So people with severe headaches get a lot of CT scans and the like, because no doctor wants to overlook a brain tumor or a brain hemorrhage. Like tension headaches, IBS is similarly defined by your symptoms—not by some lab test or X-ray exam.

Over the years experts have compiled a list of complaints that accompany IBS. In fact, the more of these complaints that

A YOUNG WOMAN WITH ABDOMINAL PAIN

Some years back I was asked to scope a young woman with stomach pain that was down low on her right side. If a patient is young, and with a typical history, most doctors diagnose IBS and begin treatment right away. National GI societies also agree with this approach. But this woman's internist told me to just humor him and do an endoscopic exam (a stomach exam) to check her for ulcers. I was certain she did not have an ulcer, but IBS. And I was dead wrong. She had two large and hard-to-miss stomach ulcers. The message here is that GI doctors often don't know what they are going to find. So if you complain enough, they will probably look "one more time."

you have, the more likely you have IBS. To give you a snapshot of the processes GI physicians use to arrive at an IBS diagnosis, here are the two schools of thought. In 1978, Manning and colleagues made a major step forward in clarifying what IBS is.[1]

MANNING CRITERIA FOR THE DIAGNOSIS OF IRRITABLE BOWEL SYNDROME*

- Pain relieved with defecation
- More frequent stools at the onset of pain
- Looser stools at the onset of pain
- Visible abdominal distention
- Passage of mucus
- Sensation of incomplete evacuation

* The likelihood of IBS is proportional to the number of Manning's criteria that are present.

An international group of IBS experts subsequently met in 1992, 1999, and again in 2005, with their primary goal being to better define IBS. At the end of each meeting, a consensus was reached describing IBS and the experts' conclusions were published as the *Rome criteria*, because the first symposium was held in Rome. So in 1992, the Rome I criteria were published; in 1999, the Rome II criteria were published; and most recently in 2005, the Rome III criteria were published. This way research in IBS could be standardized by looking at the same patient population to confirm or discredit whatever treatment was proposed for this illness. The Rome III criteria are widely considered the most up-to-date synopsis of IBS. IBS according to this classification scheme is defined by recurrent abdominal pain that occurs at least several days each month and for at least each of the preceding three months.[2] IBS should also have been a problem spanning six months or longer. Also, IBS pain is characteristically improved with passing stools, associated with a change in bowel pattern and/or change in the form (appearance) of the stool. At least two of these latter characteristics are required to secure a diagnosis of IBS in addition to pain which is a hallmark according to the Rome III criteria. Further, IBS typically has to have lasted six months or longer. More severe IBS patients have symptoms that are often daily and their illness may span years, even a decade or longer.

Not all experts fully embrace the Rome criteria, and some continue to use the Manning criteria. But the two hallmarks of IBS appear in both. The first is that the diagnosis of IBS requires recurrent abdominal pain without an identified physical cause. The second is that there is some alteration in bowel habits. Other common symptoms include nausea, reflux, indigestion,

A PATIENT WITH SEVERE IBS

Mr. H, in his midthirties, had a history of severe IBS dating back to his college years. Reviewing his thick folder of medical records, I noted that Mr. H had had numerous hospital admissions for his illness, including four admissions in the preceding year alone. In addition, he made nearly monthly trips to the emergency room. In fact, Mr. H said he did not travel anywhere without first checking in advance where the nearest hospital was located, as his attacks often coincided with trips out of town. Without fail, with each attack he would have tremendous stomach pain, explosive diarrhea, marked distention of his abdomen, and protracted vomiting. His illness typically lasted a week, but sometimes longer. By the time Mr. H came into my office, he was being followed by an internationally recognized IBS specialist at a regional university medical center.

His medical record indicated prior gallbladder surgery and an appendectomy when nothing was found during exploratory surgery. His evaluation included numerous CT scans (each abdominal CT scan has the radiation exposure of about one hundred chest X-rays!), endoscopies, colonoscopies, and so on. After all of this extensive testing, the only finding of note was mild diverticulosis of his colon. Basically, he had spent a lot of money to be probed and prodded with nothing to show for it. Anxiety and stress were thought to be contributing to his illness, and during his initial interview with me he admitted to owning a stressful business. As is common among patients with severe IBS, he was taking both antidepressant and antianxiety medications. Although anxiety and stress are thought to exacerbate IBS, research has confirmed that IBS is *not* caused by stress or anxiety problems.

Mr. H was also being followed by a well-respected gastro-enterologist in his hometown. He came to my office for a "third opinion." His father-in-law lived in the Fayetteville area and thought I might be able to help. At the time, Mr. H was taking about ten different medications for severe IBS, reflux, nausea, abdominal gas problems, and anxiety, all without much apparent benefit. One interesting remark that Mr. H offhandedly made during his first visit was that oddly, all his life he had never been able to pass gas. After reviewing his records, I gave him my "fiber talk." I also discussed why certain laxatives are beneficial in toning the colon, moving abdominal gas out of the body, and allowing the body to adapt to the fiber program. It was good that his wife was present during the interview, so that she could later reinforce my recommendations. (In my experience, often men don't follow directions nearly as well as women. And with severe IBS, following directions is key.)

Because he had been taking Citrucel for longer than a year, I told him to switch to 1 level tablespoon of Benefiber (see Chapter 3) twice daily, gradually increasing the dose to 1 well rounded tablespoon. I also told him explicitly not to use any other fiber (such as bran, oatmeal, or high-fiber cereal) until he had consistently established an excellent bathroom program. Basically he started at Week 3, Step 1 of the fiber therapy program, beginning with an intermediate dose of Benefiber because he was already on some fiber every day.

I tell all my new patients to begin at Step 1 of my fiber program if they are having abdominal gas or pain issues. It just makes good sense to use a type of fiber that is less harsh on the GI tract and that causes less gas and cramps. I also recommended that Mr. H begin Milk of Magnesia in place of the MiraLax that he had been taking. I have found that MiraLax (a synthetic laxative product) also can have a honeymoon effect; because Mr. H was having major problems on MiraLax, I thought that quite likely it was making him worse.

If Mr. H felt an impending IBS attack, he was to lie down and roll from side to side to help his excess gas move (a simple trick, but an effective maneuver for relieving gaseous discomfort following colonoscopy exams). Another suggestion to ward off an attack was that he consider using an enema in order to enable his gas to move through his system. I also warned that his IBS might initially flare up during the first couple of months of this regimen as his gut adapted to the fiber therapy program. And indeed, within the first six weeks of his initial visit, he went to the emergency room twice—but neither visit required a hospital admission. Subsequently, he has been able to stop all of his GI medicines, including his antianxiety and depression medicines, pro-motility, antispasmodic and anti-reflux medicines, and even his Zelnorm. Of note, Zelnorm (tegaserod) was a medication that was released in the U.S. for constipation and has been used for constipation predominant IBS. (More about Zelnorm later in this chapter.) I should add that Mr. H was hospitalized three times over the ensuing five years since his first visit to my office. The first time was for a GI bug that ran through his entire family and most of his office. The other two hospitalizations occurred about a year apart when he had fallen off the wagon and had dropped his fiber down to one dose each day, thinking that because he was getting good bathroom results, this was okay. All of this strongly suggests that his severe IBS is still lurking just around the corner. Indeed, at his last office visit, Mr. H remarked that in the past year he had "not had a single IBS complaint!"

A CHRISTMAS CARD FROM AN IBS PATIENT

One young woman in her early twenties, Ms. S, came in complaining of lifelong severe stomach cramps and diarrhea. I diagnosed IBS and gave her my "fiber talk." I started her on Citrucel, and her bowels promptly shut down. Within a week or so, she went from severe diarrhea to moderate constipation. After finding MiraLax an improvement over Milk of Magnesia, she sent me a card saying, "This is the best my health has been that I can ever remember." She now only takes the MiraLax if she gets into trouble, usually on one of her long road trips, and she is still following the fiber program.

I used to think that young folks would adapt fairly quickly once they embraced the program. In Ms. S's case it took several months before she began to note major improvements, even though she was following my instructions to a T. But because she was on almost weekly major road trips, her travel schedule may have offset what we were trying to achieve in the bathroom. I urged her to slow her travel schedule down and to be proactive— reminding her to step up on the laxatives before she got into the car or else shortly after she arrived at her destination. "Don't wait and let everything shut down," I reminded her.

early satiety (filling up quickly when eating just a small amount of food), distention, incomplete emptying when passing stools, lumpy or hard stools, flatulence, and frequent belching. Currently IBS is divided into three categories depending on the bowel pattern: IBS, diarrhea predominant; IBS, constipation predominant, and IBS that fluctuates between constipation and diarrhea. Scientists don't know whether these three different categories of IBS represent three distinct clinical entities or different manifestations of a single underlying disorder. I am in the second camp, and I treat all of my IBS patients using the same fiber therapy program. Further, IBS often waxes and wanes, with a wide spectrum of complaints ranging from minor periodic abdominal cramps and a few loose stools to devastating illness. Patients with IBS also make twice as many health care visits each year as their peers.[3]

Research has progressed beyond defining the illness, but not far. Today, experts talk about a paradigm shift from IBS being thought of as a *motility disorder* (I'm in the motility disorder camp, by the way) to being thought of as a *symptom-based disorder*.[4] One of the buzzwords is *visceral hypersensitivity*, which basically suggests that IBS patients respond inappropriately to everyday abdominal stress. For instance, inflating the same amount of air into an IBS patient often causes much more pain than in someone who does not have the illness. So if your doctor adheres to the visceral hypersensitivity model, he or she may tell you that there is nothing really wrong, you just have a lower pain threshold. Also, additional research indicates that IBS patients do not have appreciably more abdominal gas than healthy patients. So IBS experts have concluded that there is something wrong with IBS patients' perception of pain, leading to this visceral hypersensitivity concept. I couldn't disagree more. From my viewpoint, everyone knows that two attentive mothers will handle a crisis much differently if one has been up all night with a sick child. The research studies supporting this idea of visceral hypersensitivity are really only a single snapshot of what is actually happening inside IBS patients who have been living with their illness often for years, if not decades. To me, the person who lives with IBS for years and years is like the mother who has been up all night with a sick child. She is much more likely to snap at her children and less likely to tolerate any stress. Because gas trapping occurs much more in IBS patients, it leads to intestinal muscle spasm and therefore they are less able to tolerate any insult.

If my theory is correct, why don't IBS patients have more gas? First, abdominal gas measurements are only a radiologist's best guess based on X-ray studies. Second, and more important, because some people can tolerate constipation very well without problems, many of the "normal" control subjects likely tolerated their excess abdominal gas very nicely without ever realizing that they had a problem. For instance, I have seen a good number of patients with stomach pain who were amazed that their CT scan showed that constipation was a problem. Finally, some patients with heart failure may have a relatively normal-looking heart on chest X-ray. Also, athletes can have a heart that looks larger than normal and yet it is fine.

I had a professor at Duke University Medical School who said that it was not until the 1930s that doctors were more likely to help patients than harm them. Until then there was not much that they could really do to help; the term *patient* was used because most illnesses basically had to run their course. And these helpless doctors in the early part of the 1900s were far better physicians than those who had some newfangled cure like bloodletting, arsenic, or snake oil. Something similar is true today in the treatment of IBS. The IBS landscape is littered with promising drugs, all of which have failed to be a magic bullet for managing this disorder. Other therapies include various health products and dietary interventions, among them high-fiber and low-fiber diets, all yielding little success.

A NURSE WITH IBS AND EXPLOSIVE DIARRHEA

I remember seeing a middle-aged nurse, Mrs. Y, who came in to see me with explosive diarrhea that was so severe that at times she had loss of bowel control. Can you imagine going through life making sure you know where all the bathrooms are? Try working with a sick patient who needs your help, or being out in public at a cocktail function. Well, Mrs. Y's IBS had been going on for more than fifteen years, and she had seen two prior gastroenterologists but to no avail. Since she started the fiber therapy program, her life has improved dramatically. Almost all of you who have IBS can experience this, too, if you embrace the program.

The current focus of today's GI experts has shifted from trying to solve the IBS riddle with diet and drugs to telling patients to "be patient" and let their IBS run its course. One problem has been that to date, medications have not been terribly effective for IBS, no matter what has been tried. So IBS specialists suggest that we instead teach patients how to cope with their illness. To me, this is like trying to teach someone with pneumonia how to live with a severe cough, chest pain, and fever by giving them cooling blankets, Tylenol, and a cough suppressant without ever reaching for the needed antibiotic!

Recently I have been working with a woman with severe IBS who has not responded to the fiber therapy program. Yes, the fiber program can't help everyone, but my 90 percent success rate is a whole lot better than what is reported according to published research. At any rate, I was chatting with one of my partners about possibly referring this woman to the IBS clinic at UNC. I asked him whether any of the patients he has sent there over the years were dramatically helped. The sad answer was, "Not really." And frankly I was not surprised by his response.

Other illnesses need to be diagnosed and treated before they cause damage to the body. Yet no matter how long you've suffered, there is no apparent physical damage to the gut. So even if your IBS has been badly neglected for years if not decades, I still have success in teaching my patients how they can recover their health and their sanity. The key, once again, is marrying the program, not dabbling with fiber and not focusing on those bathroom results that are so necessary to solve your problem for good.

Functional GI Disorders (FGIDs)

IBS represents only the tip of the iceberg of "vitamin F" (fiber) deficiency. I believe that any other functional GI disorder (FGID) you can name should be lumped in the same category with IBS. FGIDs are GI disorders that leave GI doctors scratching their heads. They have no known cause and no known treatment. FGIDs include functional abdominal pain and persistent unexplained diarrhea (see Chapter 5), functional dyspepsia (indigestion and heartburnlike complaints without an identified explanation such as GE reflux and often a poor response to anti-reflux medicines such as Nexium and Prilosec), *proctalgia fugax* (fleeting but fairly severe rectal pain which has been described as feeling like a hot poker stuck up in your rectum—ouch!), and chronic bloating and gas. Typically FGIDs persist for years, their severity waxing and waning, all the while creating havoc in your life but doing no lasting

"MILK OF MAGNESIA IS YOUR FRIEND."

Mrs. T was a woman in her early seventies who had a thirty-year history of episodic diarrhea and abdominal cramps dating back to when she had lived in the Middle East for four years. She was diagnosed with some type of abdominal infection at the time, for which she received treatment, but her diarrhea and abdominal cramps had persisted ever since. I was the third GI specialist she had seen for her IBS in the previous six years. Her bowel habits varied from seven to eight loose to watery stools a day to one hard stool each day. She said that Metamucil helped her diarrhea, but she was taking it only a few times a week because it gave her so much gas. Even when she was off the Metamucil, her stomach swelled up like a beach ball, and sometimes she lost bowel control. Mrs. T's pain was in the upper abdominal area, and it got worse when she sat down. Mrs. T also complained of a second pain on the left lower side of her abdomen that was relieved with bowel movements and lying down. She also had reflux that was relatively well controlled with Prevacid. She had had an endoscopy and a colonoscopy in the year preceding her first visit to my office.

Well, Mrs. T got my "fiber talk," but it was a more expanded version because I felt it was critical to offset what her other GI doctors had told her. In addition to the usual "fiber talk," I stressed that IBS is not something you have to learn to live with. Essentially all of my IBS patients require some sort of osmotic

damage. I manage every one of them the same way I do IBS, and with approximately equal success. Of course, as with IBS, we always have to be on the lookout for other diseases that may be masquerading as an FGID.

Let's talk some about the pain characteristics of IBS and functional abdominal pain. Although the pain is generally laxative to allow them to adapt to the fiber plan, and typically this is for several months or even longer. I also tell patients, "Milk of Magnesia is your friend." That is because my patients have convinced me that constipation is at the heart of all three types of IBS disorders. If you hear *lung cancer*, you think *cigarettes*. If I hear *IBS*, I think *constipation*. For this reason, I urge all of my patients, even those complaining bitterly of explosive diarrhea, to start a laxative as soon as possible when their bowels start shutting down on the fiber program. Remember, you are not taking fiber to take fiber, you are taking fiber to get excellent bathroom results. If you don't see these results, add a laxative such as Milk of Magnesia or MiraLax to achieve that goal!

So I instructed Mrs. T to begin with Step 1 of the fiber program, stopping her Metamucil and using a synthetic fiber—Benefiber or EZ Fiber (the problem with Citrucel is that often you can find only the orange-flavored version, which makes reflux problems worse). Mrs. T was also to start Milk of Magnesia, 1–3 tablespoons daily. I told her that an added benefit was that Milk of Magnesia is an antacid, it would help with her reflux, and the magnesium was good for her bones. With this program, the diarrhea that had plagued her for more than thirty years promptly vanished, as did her stomach pains and excess abdominal gas. Her bowel control returned as well. She is now committed to the program.

located in the left lower side of the abdomen, it may involve the entire abdomen or only the upper abdomen. Generally the pain is on the left side, but for some people it is on the right side of the body. Whether it is cramping, aching, sharp, or burning, pain is the common factor in IBS. The pain may be mild or severe. It may vary from hour to hour or week to week. The pain may last from a few seconds to several hours and even all day. The pain may occur only a few days a month or even less often; at other times it occurs day in and day out. At times it may be constant for weeks or even months at a time. In essence, IBS pain and that of FGID varies tremendously. Although IBS pain may or may not be improved with passing stools or gas, it is typically associated with a change in bowel habits. Stress and food consumption frequently aggravate IBS. Other characteristics of IBS and functional abdominal pain include pain that often improves when lying down and pain occurring more commonly in the afternoon or evening. The pain may even change locations.

Remember that fever, weight loss, and rectal bleeding are uncommon with IBS. In IBS, stools may be pelletlike, ribbon-like, or loose to watery in consistency. Urgency, straining, difficulty passing stools, sensation of incomplete evacuation, and mucus are also all common complaints by people who have IBS. For IBS, the key is that one's bathroom patterns are not normal, and there is no other apparent explanation for one's stomach pain problems.

Research on Fiber in IBS

Research on the use of fiber to treat IBS was done a number of years back; these studies showed that a high-fiber diet was at best only marginally helpful, but sometimes fiber made patients worse. However, these studies were flawed because the researchers did not understand that successful treatment of IBS requires a carefully designed fiber program. These researchers just told patients to take a certain recommended dose of fiber and then recorded whether the patient's condition improved. They failed to understand that putting a patient on fiber is a process, and you cannot just suddenly start a patient on a full dose of just any type of fiber. It works much better to start with a small amount of a synthetic fiber that is less harsh on the GI tract—these cause much less gas and cramps (which is what IBS is about!)—and to proceed slowly from there. The liberal use of good-quality laxatives is also key, because almost all of these patients will require one. For this reason, the results of these studies are meaningless. Fiber cannot have a salutary effect on IBS until the body has learned to accept it and your bowels begin to move as they should.

Here is an analogy: If a blood pressure medicine does not drop your blood pressure, it will not prevent your stroke or heart attack. Similarly, if whatever fiber you take does not improve your bathroom habits, then it will not make your IBS go away. You must understand that fiber does not work like a blood pressure medicine—take it once or twice daily, and your blood pressure is under control from day one. The gut is a grouchy and sometimes unreasonable organ that has often been badly neglected for years, if not decades. It takes hard work to get the muscles of the gut moving properly again. Adding fiber to the diet or taking a fiber supplement sounds simple in theory, but often it is difficult in practice. IBS patients need to understand the reason for taking their fiber, what they are trying to achieve with the fiber, and how to get there.

Modern medicine has failed to discover that constipation and the resulting gas lock are the underlying causes of IBS. To treat IBS, you must first overcome constipation and the gas lock. This presents another problem in that most physicians, including GI specialists, do not recognize the many faces (varied presentations) of constipation. Years ago, in medical school, we were taught that syphilis was "the great imitator," masquerading as any number of different medical disorders. I believe that widespread constipation also is a great imitator. It can cause or contribute to numerous different medical problems, as described in this book (see Chapter 1). Because most doctors do not understand constipation and its association with IBS, they mention fiber only casually to the IBS patient, when fiber and laxatives should be the center of the treatment plan.

Instead, most doctors and GI specialists focus on the use of medications, including using antidepressant and antianxiety agents and also telling patients that they should learn to cope with their illness. This is not the position I take with my patients. Rather, I have the difficult job of breaking through all these misconceptions about IBS. In defense of other doctors, they have been confused by all of these flawed research studies—basically, bad research confuses everybody. In addition, fiber often makes IBS worse, especially if it is not used correctly. Thus, you can understand why doctors have focused their energies elsewhere.

Currently Available Medications for IBS

Now let's change directions and start talking about currently accepted IBS medications. Two medications for IBS—Lotronex (alosetron) and Zelnorm (tegaserod)—are only somewhat more effective than a placebo (the sugar pill) and were marketed solely to women. This means that for every ten women who take one of these medicines, only one or possibly two will be helped. Also, these medicines are incredibly expensive; Zelnorm costs $200/month if taken twice daily, and Lotronex costs $650/month. These drugs were used mostly for women because far fewer male patients participated in IBS drug studies. Because of side effects, both Zelnorm and Lotronex were recently removed temporarily from the market. They are now available again, but on a restricted basis only. Their use today is a fraction of only a few years back. One middle-aged woman walked up to me at a cocktail party and told me that she had had an IBS illness ever since childhood. When Zelnorm was taken off the market, she said she broke down and cried. Not too long thereafter, she ran across my fiber instruction sheets (I give them out by the truckload!), and she said my fiber program literally changed her life. It turned out that her husband is an attorney, and some time earlier he had helped me look into the possibility of having my three-step fiber therapy program trademarked. Knowing her dilemma and with my approval, he gave her my fiber instruction sheets. She said that she is now flying along on my program, without ever having heard my fiber spiel!

Recently, lubiprostone (Amitiza) was approved for treating women with IBS and is now available in the United States. This medicine was first used in people with constipation. Because lubiprostone is not very effective for managing constipation (see Chapter 2), I do not expect it to be very effective for IBS. Indeed, the few patients whom I have seen who were given this medicine by other physicians did not find much benefit, and several of them also had significant side effects that caused them to stop the medicine.

Bacterial Overgrowth of the Small Bowel, Antibiotics, and Probiotics

Recently, research in IBS has focused on a condition called *bacterial overgrowth* as possibly causing or heavily contributing to IBS illnesses. The healthy small intestine is virtually sterile with only a few bacteria present. Your stomach acid kills most bacteria that you ingest, so that digestion of your food occurs normally. Research studies suggest that bacterial overgrowth of the small intestine can cause abdominal pain and alterations in bowel habits due to maldigestion of your food—an IBS-like illness. There are currently two camps: researchers who think that overgrowth of bacteria in the small bowel causes much of the IBS symptoms, and those who think that bacterial overgrowth represents at most only a small subset of IBS patients. At this point, research is not conclusive. The problem stems in part from the difficulty of determining whether this condition is present. One way to diagnose bacterial overgrowth is to run a scope into the mouth and through the esophagus and stomach, collecting fluid from the small intestines. This is expensive and not always accurate, as the mouth and esophagus are not sterile, so the fluid that is collected may be contaminated. Another way is to have the patient swallow a sugar such as glucose or lactulose, and if there are too many bacteria in the small intestine, they ferment the sugars, releasing hydrogen gas. Breath hydrogen can then be measured when the patient exhales. Unfortunately, these tests are also not as accurate as we would like.

If you are in the first camp and believe that bacterial overgrowth of the small bowel commonly occurs and causes an IBS-like illness, then finding the right antibiotic or *probiotic* (live bacteria that are eaten; they are thought to establish healthier gut flora) could be a solution for solving the IBS puzzle. Indeed, certain antibiotics such as rifaximin appear promising, and some patients appear to improve at least for a number of months. However, antibiotics do not address the underlying reason as to why bacterial overgrowth occurs in the first place. Patients with IBS should expect to require periodic courses of antibiotics for the rest of their lives. And of course, antibiotics have problems of their own, such as allergic reactions and antibiotic resistance. In fact, a few of my patients with difficult cases of IBS have tried antibiotics, and in my mind the jury is still out as to whether there was any real benefit.

Probiotics are considered relatively harmless and in some respects more "natural." They are found in certain brands of yogurt and fermented milk and also in pills. Unfortunately, this is an unregulated industry. So just about anyone can make whatever claim they wish and not be challenged by any regulatory agency, the FDA included. Another problem is that there are a growing number of different types of probiotics, and which is best for you? However, because these products are thought to be harmless, it is reasonable to try one to see if it helps. I cannot make any suggestions here as to what product to use other than selecting a product distributed by a well-known manufacturer. Companies such as Dannon make every effort to ensure that their product is safe, but efficacy is another matter. Once again, there is a lot of hype, and whatever you read today about probiotics, ten years from now the information will likely be quite different as there is a lot of ongoing research in this area. Read the labels. Because efficacy is an unknown at this point for probiotics, safety of whatever product you select should be a high priority.

But here again, researchers in probiotics have forgotten to ask the basic question as to why bacterial overgrowth occurs in the first place. As with reflux and gas problems, if you don't address the underlying problem, you will not have a long-term solution for the problem. If bacterial overgrowth does occur, I expect that a weak ileocecal valve (the sphincter muscle at the end of the small intestine that relaxes to allow undigested food waste to move through to the colon) would be the likely cause. Impaired muscle contractions of the bowel (also caused by constipation) causing stasis is a second explanation. Since your food is not swept out of your body as it should be, whatever few bacteria are in your small intestines (recall that even in healthy people the small intestines have a few bacteria) begin multiplying, changing your small bowel from a pond into a cesspool. Not a pretty picture, I know. But why else should some people get bacterial overgrowth (if indeed this occurs)? Either way, long-standing constipation impairs bowel motility (recall that your gut is one long tube, and what happens at one end will affect what happens at the other end because there is a single pacemaker in the stomach) and thereby contributes to the conditions predisposing you to intestinal bacterial overgrowth. So from this vantage point, if your constipation problem is never addressed, whatever agent is used to solve this problem I expect will ultimately fail. At most, my belief is that probiotics and antibiotics may at best one day play a supporting role in the management of IBS. In that situation, if patients are not responding to the fiber therapy program, then a course of probiotics or antibiotics may be considered. Probiotics may also help prevent relapses—serving as a security blanket, if you will—when for whatever reason you can't keep your GI tract making those necessary bathroom stops as it should.

A Few Other Notes on IBS

The older medication classes such as TCAs (tricyclic antidepressants), SSRIs (selective serotonin reuptake inhibitors), and antispasmodics are marginal at best in relieving the symptoms of IBS, and some evidence even suggests that antispasmodics can make IBS worse. I don't like antispasmodics (and Lotronex for the same reason) because they have a constipating effect. In an individual patient, one of these medicines may be helpful, but most folks do not obtain significant long-term help from any prescribed medication for IBS. However, a few of my patients are on one product or other because for them the fiber therapy program does not control their complaints completely. For instance, among my patients I have a middle-aged woman who is taking a low dose of amitriptyline at bedtime, and also a nurse in her thirties who takes nortriptyline as needed (these are the only two patients in my practice who take these medicines). Both women closely follow the fiber therapy program and use these products adjunctively. But most physicians have found that these medicines are not a general solution for IBS problems, nor do I expect the latest up-and-coming medicine (whatever that may be) to be a cure-all either.

Again, I believe that it doesn't make horse sense to use a chemical agent to solve a mechanical problem. If your drain has a major blockage, Drano (your pills) may help loosen the stuff up, but you still need a plunger (good-quality synthetic fiber that won't cause a lot of gas and make the problem worse) and often "the snake" (those long metal rods that plumbers use; in our example, laxatives such as Milk of Magnesia, MiraLax, and prunes and prune juice and even enemas) to open up your pipes. Also, stopped-up plumbing systems have a bad odor, just like your GI tract when you get into trouble. Remember that your gut is one thirty-foot-long muscle. Pills such as Zelnorm, Amitiza, or Lotronex are just not going to get your gut (which has gotten spastic over a number of years and is doing only the minimum of what it needs to do) working as it should. It just won't happen, no matter how many pills or what kinds of pills you pour into your system. And unlike the blocked drain, one good plunge or one pass of the snake generally won't do the job because it is not six inches of your gut that is a problem, but more likely than not five to ten feet or more of your intestines that are not working as they should.

I can't say too often that this process has to overcome months, if not years, of neglect. It takes time, and you have to stay focused on making certain that your gut does what it needs to do every day in the bathroom. In the old days it wasn't much of a problem. Just about everybody worked hard for a living; they also ate high-quality grains, did not sleep in on the weekends, and certainly didn't travel a hundred miles at the drop of a hat. Knowing what good bowel habits were was common knowledge to everyone (and even doctors) back then! If you got a little slow, you reached for an apple or prunes. But you didn't sit around on your thumbs hoping that things would be back on track the next day, or the next week for that matter.

Today we remember the saying, "An apple a day keeps the doctor away," but not what it actually meant. Because people back then had well-toned systems, an apple or two or a few prunes was all it took to jump-start your bathroom results when they slowed down. Not so today. People wait until they have severe constipation problems before they ever think about doing something different. This is a big mistake. Whenever I travel or sleep in on the weekends, I give my fiber program a little help by eating nuts (which are high in magnesium) or an apple (my preference). For you it could be Milk of Magnesia or MiraLax. Anyway, this is so important that I felt it necessary to reiterate this key message.

Years back, in the middle of the night, our then-twelve-year-old daughter, Rosie, came upstairs crying because of severe stomach pain. At first I thought that she might have appendicitis, so severe was her pain. But her abdomen was okay and she didn't have a fever. Sure enough, this was the beginning of a long saga with IBS. At times she had severe cramps and diarrhea, and even reflux and vomiting. Sometimes she just could not get out of the bathroom. Now kids you have to handle with special gloves, especially your only daughter. Over the years Rosie had periodic flare-ups of IBS, but this was because she never fully bought into her father's program. She took her fiber only erratically, never having the necessary bathroom results that are so critical to managing this problem.

This past fall, Rosie did a study abroad in Quito, Ecuador, and got into big-time IBS trouble with stomach pain and going back and forth between severe diarrhea and constipation.

She could not get her bowels regulated by drinking loads of prune juice, taking Milk of Magnesia, and drinking coffee with Benefiber. In part this was due to all of her traveling around the countryside. As a last resort, we shipped a large can of Citrucel to her via FedEx, praying that customs would let this container go through. Sure enough, she overcame the gas lock problem that I assumed she had. The problem was that the Benefiber she had been taking for some time had lost its advantage (the honeymoon effect was gone) and was causing as much gas as if she had been on Metamucil or bran. In the wake of this experience, for the first time Rosie really listened, especially because I told her that the problem would almost certainly again return even on Citrucel if she did not adhere to the program. A frank discussion ensued about not selling out and not backing off laxatives until stellar bathroom results were consistently achieved; up until then she had only paid lip service to this idea. Now she is flying and has never looked back. She is off the Citrucel and on bran and Metamucil and doing fabulously for the first time ever. Why? Because she finally fully bought into the program, becoming fearless when it came to using MiraLax or Milk of Magnesia to get her going that extra mile.

Unfortunately, Rosie had a setback this spring. She immediately went back to Citrucel, and she also resumed MiraLax and prunes. But this time her GI tract did not respond as it had last fall. After another several weeks, she finally called and alerted me to her dilemma. I used the example of the Duke basketball team playing UNC in a season-ending title game. If Duke is down by ten points in the first five minutes of play, Coach K will adjust his strategy and probably also his players on the court. After he makes the changes, he does not wait until well into the second half of the game to make another change. No, Coach K is constantly tweaking his team as best he can to gain the advantage. The point I made to Rosie was that it was great and all that she went back to the Citrucel, prunes, and MiraLax when she got into trouble, but if a week passes without much progress, she needs to do something else rather than waiting several weeks. We lost a lot of ground in the process. For her, this meant switching over to EZ Fiber, and I urged her to use a magnesium product, preferably Milk of Magnesia or magnesium citrate (because the tablets are not as effective). She got much better results the next day and is now making good progress again.

Recall that MiraLax also has a honeymoon effect, and so it can be counterproductive when a gas lock situation develops. However, bacteria cannot ferment metals well, so this honeymoon effect is not a problem with the magnesium products. If these adjustments do not take effect, then try to work from below with a glycerin suppository, a Fleet enema, or, if worse comes to worst, a tap-water enema. The comment here? Desperate people do desperate things. If pushing from above is not working, sometimes it's best to pull from below.

The Three-Step Fiber Program for People with IBS

The treatment program for IBS is basically the same as the three-step program in Chapter 3. Remember that one hat fits everyone. Unfortunately, space constraints do not allow us to have the same detailed look at the fiber plan here for IBS patients as we had in Chapter 3. But rest assured that in my office, I give the same fiber instruction sheets to my IBS patients as to everyone else. Rather, this section will broadly review the fiber therapy program and highlight areas of particular interest for people with IBS.

STEP 1

Step 1 is easy: Take ½ tablespoon of Citrucel, Benefiber, or EZ Fiber twice daily. If you are afraid of fiber because of a past bad experience, 1 level teaspoon twice daily would be a good idea. If you have excess gas or cramps with one fiber product, try a different one. The important thing about this step is to get into the habit of taking your fiber twice daily; each week, try taking a little more, building up to 1 well-rounded tablespoon twice daily over the next four to six weeks. So if in Week 1 you chose to start with 1 level teaspoon of fiber twice daily, in Week 2 you should take 1 rounded teaspoon twice daily. Then in Week 3, take ¾ of a tablespoon twice daily. And in Week 4, take 1 level tablespoon twice daily. Week 5 would be 1 slightly rounded tablespoon twice daily; finally, in Week 6, take 1 heaping tablespoon twice daily. (Also note that if you are using Citrucel with sugar, you would start with ½ tablespoon and build up to 1½ scoops or 3 level tablespoons twice daily over the same five-to-six-week interval). Leave your fiber container out on the countertop so that you won't forget to take your fiber. Remember, I use a different amount of fiber than what the manufacturers recommend.

Benefiber caplets and Citrucel capsules may be substituted for the powdered products. For Step 1 of Week 1, you would start with 1 Benefiber caplet twice daily (or this could be 1 Citrucel capsule twice daily). Each week you would take an additional Benefiber caplet or Citrucel capsule: So for Week 2, this would be 2 twice daily; for Week 3, 3 twice daily; for Week 4, 4 twice daily; and for Week 5, 5 twice daily. The maximum daily dose of Benefiber caplets would be 5 twice daily (ten daily), but for Citrucel capsules you are to build up to 6 twice daily (twelve), which would be Week 6 of Step 1. Make sure that you don't mistake the psyllium capsules as being equivalent to Benefiber or Citrucel. They are not and may cause much cramping, especially if you have IBS. For those on a limited budget, there is a generic brand for Benefiber (wheat dextrin) and Citrucel (methylcellulose).

If you were already eating a bowl of bran flakes before starting the three-step fiber program, or perhaps taking a dose of Metamucil most days, I suggest that for now you stop your bran or Metamucil and use a midrange dose of the synthetic fiber, such as ¾ of a tablespoon or even 1 level tablespoon twice daily (this would be two or three Benefiber caplets or Citrucel capsules). This would mean starting at Week 2 or 3 of Step 1 of the fiber therapy program. Also, during Step 1, it is often necessary to give your colon "a daily push" with a laxative such as Milk of Magnesia or magnesium tablets, prunes or prune juice, or MiraLax or GlycoLax. One point I need to make very clear: Using a laxative is almost uniformly necessary for my IBS patients. So if you have IBS and no matter how much diarrhea you think you have, know that very shortly you will need a laxative once you start the fiber therapy program. It's hard to believe, but true. Of course, if you have IBS and constipation and gas are major problems for you, then start the laxative as soon as you start Step 1 rather than waiting to add it later on. But because all folks with IBS, including those with diarrhea, are constipated, it is the rule rather than the exception that you will need a laxative for your gut to adapt to the fiber therapy program. So don't be afraid! Take your laxative daily if you need it, and I am fairly certain that you will.

I need to stop for a moment to throw out a word of caution. Patients with IBS often experience flare-ups of their illness when they first get on the fiber program. I know that I told you this earlier in the chapter, but some things need to be clearly spelled out, and this is one of them. All fiber sources, to a greater or lesser degree, can start fermenting in your large intestine. In the early stages of the fiber program, your GI tract is not yet moving as well as it should. Thus, when you first start the program, your fiber stays in contact with bacteria longer than you want, creating a potential of excess gas—even if you are using one of the newer synthetic fiber products. This is why using a laxative early on in the process with my IBS patients is so important. Gas and spasm are what cause your pain, and by ingesting fiber, you will have more gas. If you have a muscle cramp in your leg, it hurts worse when you stretch it. So it is with IBS. So you want to get the fiber in and out of your system as soon as possible. But if you are having more pain than is usual for you, get yourself checked out by your health care provider to be certain that everything is okay. Also consider going back to Week 1 of the fiber program, and if there is still a problem, perhaps switching to a different fiber product (e.g. if you were having too many problems with Benefiber, you might want to try Citrucel, or vice versa).

Once your bowels begin moving efficiently, the problem of excess gas should subside. This is why it is so important to accelerate your bowels' processing of the leftovers and pushing them out of your body as quickly as possible by using a good-quality laxative and being selective about which new synthetic fiber you choose. A gas lock may occur with anyone who takes fiber for the first time, but it tends to be more severe for those with IBS (they are the ones who have the grouchy, unreasonable colons that complain at the drop of a hat) and especially if you are using the wrong kind of fiber, which is immediately recognized by your gut bacterial flora and attacked. You just want to minimize that fermentation process (think putrefaction) inside of you as much as possible. And the only way to do this is to get everything moving on through and out as soon as possible.

STEP 2

In Step 2, you will begin expanding your diet to what I consider overall better-quality fiber products. You should have been on Step 1 for at least four to six weeks, and you should advance to this step only if you are making several excellent bathroom stops each day. For most of my patients, it takes at least several weeks and often a few months to achieve those excellent bathroom stops. Another key with Steps 1 and 2 is patience. Don't try to rush the process. Stay on top of your bowels, don't back off, and keep nudging them to act several times daily with good results. Small pieces of stool several times a day doesn't count. We are talking cow poop (or at least some semblance thereof). My apologies to those of you who are offended by my having to be so graphic, but I really have to spell this out once again, since this is of utmost importance for my IBS patients. Remember that less-than-sweet odor, excess gas, noisy stomachs, frequent belching, reflux, and small stools are also signs of constipation. It is when you can't believe what is happening in the bathroom that you can begin thinking about moving from Step 1 to Step 2 and decreasing your laxative dose. A forty-year-old couch potato just cannot decide to go out and run in a ten-kilometer race after only a couple of weeks of training. Your colon has been living a couch potato lifestyle, typically for decades, and it is going to take weeks if not months of regular bathroom stops before it is capable of moving to Step 2.

Step 2 really serves as a bridge to Step 3. In Step 2 you cut your synthetic fiber dose in half to 1 level tablespoon of sugar-free Citrucel, Benefiber, or EZ Fiber (or this would be 3 Benefiber caplets or 3 Citrucel capsules) for breakfast, and you have a cup of oatmeal or bran flakes. Or you may have 2 slices of a high-quality whole-wheat bread plus 1 level tablespoon of Citrucel, Benefiber, or EZ Fiber for breakfast. See Chapter 3 for more specific details. Another option would be to take 1 rounded teaspoon of sugar-free Metamucil (a half-serving of Metamucil as I measure it) with your half-dose of Benefiber. The reason why I don't want you to go from Step 1 to Step 3, skipping Step 2 in the process, is that your intended bathroom results may not be as settled as they really ought to be. So test the waters before moving on to Step 3, to get an idea of how well your GI tract will tolerate what I consider better-quality fiber. If your bathroom stops are not what they should be, stomach cramps and even a gas lock may become a problem. If that is the case, go back to Step 1 and wait a bit longer. Perhaps also you should increase your laxative dose a little. Take your time. Some folks find that they just prefer to stay on Week 5 or 6 of Step 1 indefinitely; this is fine as long as you continue to get those satisfactory bathroom results that are so necessary to keep your IBS at bay.

STEP 3

Now, on to Step 3. If your excellent bathroom results have been pretty consistent for at least several weeks on Step 2, and if your stools are bulky and soft, with minimal odor, and gas is not much of an issue, only now can you consider stopping your Citrucel, Benefiber, or EZ Fiber entirely and move on to a full dose of psyllium (Metamucil, Konsyl, Fiberall, Hydrocil) and/ or entirely to high-quality fiber foods. You could stay indefinitely with a synthetic fiber product such as Citrucel, Benefiber, or EZ Fiber, but because I haven't found them quite as effective as the rest of the pack, you will not likely be able to wean off your laxatives as easily. If you choose to go to Step 3, make sure that you are consistently maintaining those excellent bathroom results that are so key to controlling your IBS. If not, consider upping your dose of laxative, or even going back to Step 1 if you are having issues with the program. There will be false starts along the way. It's like riding a bicycle. Sometimes you just have to go back to the training wheels (Step 1) for a while until everything settles down and you are comfortable with the program.

Expanding Your Food and Medication Boundaries

I can't begin to count how many people have told me that they just can't eat certain foods, and especially salads and cucumbers.

The idea here is that with your GI tract working as it should, everything just keeps moving down your pipes. Pills don't just sit forever in your stomach, because everything is being swept through with excellent gut peristalsis. However, if your system is not well tuned, then everything changes. The little extra gas that you get with eating raw vegetables such as lettuce and cucumbers becomes an issue because your gas is not moving through as it should and your GI tract is just too rigid to accommodate the small additional gas load, or you may

A MAN WHO COULDN'T EAT LETTUCE

One stocky man in his midforties told me, "I can't even eat the lettuce on a hamburger; it just tears my stomach up to no end!" I told him that his intolerance of lettuce was a sign that he probably had a lurking IBS problem, even though he said his bowel habits were fine. The problem was that what little gas he got from eating lettuce stayed trapped inside him and just wouldn't move through as it should. Once he established better bathroom habits, he would be just fine, because his gut would tolerate the little extra gas that lettuce causes. Sure enough, in just six short weeks, he returned smiling and announced, "I can now eat a small garden salad without any problems!" I remarked that soon he would be eating a chef's salad if he continued on the fiber therapy program.

A YOUNG WOMAN WHO COULD NOT TAKE ANTIBIOTICS

Another patient, a young woman in her twenties, walked into my office for a second opinion because she could not tolerate the antibiotics that were prescribed for her *H. pylori* stomach infection (which predisposes the patient to ulcers and possibly stomach cancer), which was found during an endoscopy done by another GI doctor. Ms. N had tried three different times to take the antibiotics, but she would get very ill with severe cramps and vomiting within a matter of hours. Sure enough, she had a mild case of IBS, which up until then had not been diagnosed. Once we got her GI tract working as it should and getting her IBS under better control, I thought she might be able to tolerate those antibiotics better. So this time, after six months of the fiber therapy program, she took the entire two-week course of antibiotics without so much as a hiccup.

even have a gas lock situation without even knowing it. Like many medicines, antibiotics are tough on your stomach, especially if they just sit there for hours before moving on down the pike. However, if your GI tract is moving everything along as it should, you will have much fewer problems tolerating all those foods that you couldn't eat before, and that includes tolerating medicines such as antibiotics.

This is one of the truly remarkable things about the fiber program: People are often surprised, and at times even amazed, at what they can now eat. Indeed, once you have fully adapted to the fiber therapy program and are making several excellent bathroom stops daily, you will probably be able to eat and enjoy, without fear, many of the foods that had given you trouble.

KEY POINTS TO REMEMBER

- Most people do not have to learn to live with their IBS!

- IBS may be worsened by stress, but stress does not cause IBS.

- Most IBS patients can stop taking their IBS medications once their gut is well adapted to the fiber therapy program.

- The fiber therapy program used to treat IBS is the same three-step program outlined in Chapter 3. Almost all of my IBS patients will require a laxative at first as their body adapts to the fiber, and this is often for at least several months, even if diarrhea was the main problem.

- IBS may flare up when you start the fiber program, so go slowly.

- Be proactive! Stay on top of your bowels. Don't give them an inch. Anticipate problems and make an adjustment if needed. Use a glycerin suppository or enema if necessary. See your health care provider if you are not making progress or are getting worse.

- The fiber therapy program will often expand your horizons to include foods and medications you couldn't tolerate before.

Notes

1. Manning AP, Thompson WG, Heaton KW, Morris AF. Towards positive diagnosis of the irritable bowel. *Br Med J.* 1978;2(6138):653–654.

2. Longstreth GF, Thompson WG, Chey WD, Houghton LA, Mearin F, Spiller RC. Functional bowel disorders. *Gastroenterology.* 2006;130:1480–1491.

3. Levy RL, Whitehead WE, Von Korff MR, Feld AD. Intergenerational transmission of gastrointestinal illness behavior. *Am J Gastroenterol.* 2000;95:451–456.

4. Drossman, DA. What does the future hold for irritable bowel syndrome and the functional gastrointestinal disorders? *J Clin Gastroenterol.* 2005;39(suppl 3):S251–S256.

CHAPTER 8

Taming Crohn's Disease, Ulcerative Colitis, Celiac Sprue, and Diverticulosis

Most physicians, and especially gastroenterologists, would find it odd to include these four relatively diverse illnesses in a book about fiber. In particular, Crohn's disease, ulcerative colitis, and celiac sprue are considered largely inflammatory disorders of the bowel, and if you open a textbook of medicine concerning any one of these diseases, it will not mention fiber as being beneficial. It will, however, include a lot of information about inflammation or colitis (-*itis* means inflammation, as in *appendicitis, arthritis,* and *bursitis*). Medical textbooks focus solely on the various therapies for the inflammatory component of the illness, and for those with sprue the discussion centers on dietary restriction of gluten. Admittedly, diverticulosis is thought to be related to deficient dietary fiber, at least by most authorities. Recently, however, a small cohort of GI experts has become increasingly vocal in noting that irritable bowel syndrome (IBS) often coexists in patients with Crohn's disease and ulcerative colitis. I wholeheartedly agree. I

believe that all of these disorders are a tip-off that we are deal-
ing with not just a problem of inflammation, but also a problem
with insufficient fiber in the diet and unrecognized consti-
pation. Almost all of my patients with one of these disorders
eventually embrace the three-step fiber program to manage
their bowel complaints, when they realize that their urgency,
cramps, gas problems, and such can indeed be helped.

In essence, even though the inflammatory component of
your Crohn's disease or ulcerative colitis may be under good
control, you may still have the same symptoms that led to
your initial diagnosis: diarrhea, urgency, stomach cramps, and
abdominal gas. If so, I believe that your symptoms are no lon-
ger due to inflammation (because it is under control according
to your GI doctor), but rather due to underlying and untreated
IBS. Ten percent of IBS patients report experiencing some kind
of acute gastroenteritis that precipitated the beginning of their
troubles, eventually leading to their diagnosis of IBS. Like a
person with an acute GI bug that never seems to go away and is
eventually recognized as IBS, some patients with Crohn's dis-
ease or ulcerative colitis just can't seem to shake their illness
even when it appears to be under control as determined by a
colonoscopy or lab tests. Whether the patient has Crohn's dis-
ease, ulcerative colitis, sprue, or some other GI problem, the
real problem is the incipient IBS that causes all kinds of mis-
chief, and yet nobody ever suspects what is actually happening.

Like patients who have been diagnosed with IBS, those
diagnosed with Crohn's disease, ulcerative colitis, or sprue have
also been told that though medication may alleviate some of
their symptoms, they will need to learn to live with their illness.
My job then is doubly hard, because I have to break through

this mind-set that everything is due to inflammation. *I can't say it too loudly: If your Crohn's disease or ulcerative colitis is found to be in remission by a colonoscopy (that is, if no inflammation is evident) or by whatever tests are done to assess your problems, then your Crohn's disease or ulcerative colitis is no longer the problem causing your persistent symptoms.* Keep taking your medicines, but shift your attention to the IBS that until now has not been recognized. If this is news to you, and if you don't know what IBS is, go back and read Chapter 7 before proceeding.

I have been told that in China, the physician is not paid if the patient does not get better. Perhaps if doctors in the United States were held accountable in a similar manner, physicians would do a better job. Too many physicians order a test or prescribe a medication to get their patients out the door, without ever really sitting down and helping them figure out what may really improve their lives. One family physician once told me that he "just kept ordering tests" until the patient stopped complaining! Sad but an all too often true statement concerning the state of our health care system.

If you find that your doctor only treats the inflammatory condition of your Crohn's disease, ulcerative colitis, celiac sprue, or diverticulosis and does not address the underlying IBS, you may find yourself trading the symptoms of one illness (Crohn's disease, ulcerative colitis, sprue, or diverticulosis) for another (IBS). By no means does this chapter intend to suggest that the inflammatory disorders of Crohn's disease or ulcerative colitis can be managed without medications, nor will the patient with celiac disease be able to eat food containing gluten without problems. The point I want you to take away is that just controlling your inflammatory bowel disorder with medications or your sprue with diet is often only half the battle, and more often than not this will not solve all of your problems.

Crohn's Disease

Crohn's disease is an inflammatory condition of the entire wall of your bowel. It can affect any portion of the gastrointestinal tract from your mouth all the way down to your rectum and anus. This makes it uniquely different from ulcerative colitis, which affects only the inner lining of the large intestine. Although Crohn's disease and ulcerative colitis are considered different disorders, there is considerable overlap in both their symptoms and their management. Sometimes your doctor won't be able to tell which condition you have because at colonoscopy, Crohn's disease and ulcerative colitis may look exactly the same.

The causes of both disorders are unknown (what doctors call *idiopathic*: *idio-* meaning we don't know, and *-pathic* meaning we wish we did). Blood tests may help distinguish one disorder from the other—but again, not always. Both conditions are also associated with a rare liver disorder called *sclerosing cholangitis* (which may lead to liver failure and even need for a liver transplant) and increased risk for developing intestinal cancer. Both Crohn's disease and ulcerative colitis have also been associated with arthritis, mouth ulcers, a skin condition called *pyoderma gangrenosum* (with a name like that you know it must look terrible), *erythema nodosum* (another skin disorder that comes and goes), and even ocular lesions. Many of the medicines used to treat Crohn's disease are also used to treat ulcerative colitis.

But there are also distinct differences between Crohn's disease and ulcerative colitis. Crohn's disease commonly causes strictures, fibrous bands of scar tissue that narrow the small intestine, sometimes causing a bowel obstruction, and thereby may require surgery. (In ulcerative colitis, strictures that cause symptoms are rare). Crohn's disease can also cause fistulas (contained ruptures of the bowel wall), which are caused by severe inflammation forming penetrating ulcers that erode completely through the bowel wall, at times ending blindly and causing an abscess. These fistulas may even tunnel into other organs such as the urinary bladder, the vagina, or even outside the body through the skin. Fortunately, most patients with Crohn's disease do not develop fistulas or strictures.

Other hallmarks of Crohn's disease include fever, weight loss, anemia, abdominal pain, and diarrhea, often with bleeding. In children and adolescents, an early tip-off is growth retardation, in which the child suddenly stops growing. This may be his or her only symptom. The abdominal pain may be brief hard cramps or longer and continuous pain. The pain usually affects the entire abdomen but may also be localized to one principal area, usually but not always the right lower abdomen.

Oddly, smoking seems to help ulcerative colitis. A few years back, our group admitted a middle-aged man with a severe flare-up of ulcerative colitis who had recently stopped smoking. Our debate centered on whether it would be best for him to resume smoking in order to help get his colitis under control. We tried the nicotine patch but to no avail. Now that is a dire strait, when a doctor recommends smoking for someone's health!

But the reverse is true with patients with Crohn's disease. I strongly discourage smoking, not just for my patients with Crohn's disease, but I also ask that their spouses stop smoking as well. I even recommend that my patients request a smoke-free area when dining out at a restaurant. My most problematic patients with Crohn's disease are those who continue smoking. It is remarkable that when patients really understand that their Crohn's disease is made worse by smoking, many of them are able to quit. To my knowledge, every review of Crohn's disease emphatically states that controlling the illness is hampered if patients choose to continue smoking. Eventually, I have succeeded in getting all of my patients with Crohn's disease to stop (at least that is what they tell me!).

Birth control pills were once reported to also cause flare-ups of Crohn's disease, but after careful study it seems that only birth control pills that have high estrogen and progesterone may worsen the illness. These pills are sometimes prescribed in Europe. But in the United States all birth control pills are low dose and are no longer considered a contraindication for women who have Crohn's disease.

One underappreciated aspect of Crohn's is the business of milk allergy. We are not talking lactose intolerance, but rather that something in milk products seems to exacerbate Crohn's disease. Perhaps it is an allergy to lactose, or perhaps some protein in milk is creating the problem.

A BUSINESSMAN WITH CROHN'S
AND DIARRHEA

Mr. Z was a fifty-year-old businessman with a forty-year history of Crohn's disease when he came to see me. He had been treated by GI physicians across the United States and even at the Mayo Clinic. He told me that since the onset of his illness, he had regularly taken twenty or more Lomotil or Imodium tablets each week, and yet still he had only partial control of his bowels. Urgency also was a major problem, especially when he played golf. (Urgency means that you have to suddenly rush to do your business in the bathroom, and if you delay by more than a moment or two you may not make it. If you have major cramps as well, doctors call it *tenesmus*.) Playing golf could become a particularly embarrassing situation for him because everybody in his foursome could not help but notice how many bathroom stops he was making during their four-hour round of golf. At any rate, we did a colonoscopy and found moderately active colitis, with irregular linear ulcers that were characteristic of Crohn's disease. I started Mr. Z on 6-MP (mercaptopurine, a weak chemotherapy-type drug used for inflammatory bowel and other noncancerous disorders). From his first visit to the office, I also began encouraging Mr. Z to add some fiber to his diet, telling him that this would probably help much of his diarrhea, stomach cramps, and urgency complaints.

Mr. Z was a busy executive who was quite skeptical from the start about my fiber regimen, especially because no prior GI physician, including those at the Mayo Clinic, had made this recommendation. Quite often when patients have been talking with their doctors for years about their condition, they come to feel that they have a better handle on it and are nearly experts on it themselves. Mr. Z knew, too, that fiber is a laxative, and this was the last thing he thought he needed. Though none of the GI specialists he had been treated by had come close to improving his condition, I could tell that he wasn't really taking my advice seriously. Basically, he wanted me to keep filling his prescription for the Lomotil. I understood that. Why in the world should he take something that was guaranteed to make his problems worse? This went on for several years and there really wasn't much more I could do. But after numerous visits to my office and hearing my broken record play my fiber song again and again, he grudgingly began to add some high-quality fiber to his diet. I should add that I was helped in this by a couple of his business acquaintances who were also patients of mine. They kept harping on him as well to get on with the fiber program if he ever wanted to get better.

At first he took only one dose of fiber daily, but eventually when he saw that it didn't increase his diarrhea and actually was helping, he increased it to twice daily. He always seemed to settle for less than stellar results, largely because whatever was happening in the bathroom was so much better than what had ever been happening before. Once he finally committed to the full fiber program, he became a staunch advocate. His complaints of urgency, stomach pain, loss of bowel control, and diarrhea eventually disappeared. He now rarely if ever takes Imodium or Lomotil. Also, he recently commented how much more he now enjoys golf since he no longer has to make all those bathroom stops as in past years.

A CROHN'S PATIENT WITH SEVERE MILK ALLERGY

Fifteen years back, there was a medical report of a man with severe Crohn's disease who was dependent on prednisone, and yet he still had moderately active Crohn's disease with pain and diarrhea. He also had had two surgical procedures for his diseased bowel, yet his Crohn's disease remained active. Someone eventually suggested that he get off milk products entirely, and in a matter of several months he was able to stop taking all of his medicines, including his prednisone.

Two years later, he and his physician decided to do a small scientific experiment to determine whether milk was in fact the culprit. He was given a can of Ensure (a food supplement that is milk free) to drink three times a day for three days. The doctor was going to put two teaspoons of milk in the Ensure, but he was not going to tell him when he was doing it. The patient did very well the first two days. But on the third day his doctor added two teaspoons of milk. Within an hour or so of his morning dose, the patient began having stomach cramps and diarrhea that lasted a good bit of the morning. When lunchtime arrived, he refused to drink the second can of Ensure.

I don't wish to belabor the point, but I think people with Crohn's disease really need to understand that milk products can make their symptoms much worse, perhaps on the same order of magnitude as smoking. Sometimes the reaction won't occur for two or three days and it may be very insidious, not nearly as dramatic as described earlier. So I tell my patients that just because they don't think they have a problem with

A CROHN'S PATIENT WHO HAD EMERGENCY SURGERY

One of my patients was a young man who was built like a football player. After he was hospitalized for a flare-up of his Crohn's disease, accompanied by high fever and severe stomach pain with bleeding, I convinced him to stop all milk products entirely. Several months after he got out of the hospital, I received a call that he was headed back to the emergency room once again with severe stomach pain and high fever. He was operated on later that week for peritonitis from a bowel perforation linked to his Crohn's disease. He later told me that he had so dearly missed drinking milk that one morning he just swished some milk in his mouth only an hour or so before having to rush to the hospital.

milk, they cannot afford to be mistaken. Crohn's can cause a very serious illness. I estimate that almost all of my Crohn's patients heed this advice and they themselves come to this same conclusion that milk products can definitely cause flares of their illness. The best thing to do is to get off milk products for several months and then if you are doing well, you might give yourself a test dose of say a teaspoon of milk. Don't decide that day. See how you do that week. But be forewarned that your Crohn's may flare if you try this (see page 206).

Before the arrival of agents such as Remicade (infliximab) and Humira (adalimumab), experts generally believed that 50 percent of patients with Crohn's disease would require surgery roughly every seven years. In fact, twenty years ago, one of our goals of treatment was to delay surgery as long as

A CROHN'S PATIENT WHO INSISTED
ON DRINKING MILK

I once saw a patient in his sixties who was convinced that milk was just what he needed, and he drank several glasses every day. He wouldn't dream of touching Ensure or Boost. As ill as he was, you would have thought that he might have tried to lay off milk even for a couple of weeks just to see if by any chance his severe diarrhea and bleeding might be related. But some people just never listen, and he paid a steep price for being hardheaded when a severe attack of Crohn's disease proved fatal.

possible, because after two or three operations, the concern was that patients might lose so much of their bowel that they would require TPN (total parenteral nutrition; being fed intravenously), because a severely shortened bowel would not be able to absorb enough nutrition for survival.

Remicade and Humira have changed all of this. Both are considered biologic agents in that they alter the immune response, thereby controlling the illness. These are powerful drugs, and serious and possibly life-threatening infections may accompany their use. They are also terribly expensive, costing about $20,000 annually. So although Remicade and Humira are considered lifesavers for many patients with Crohn's disease, most GI physicians use them only as a last resort. In recent years, some experts have argued that physicians should use these agents early if the patient's illness is severe, saying that it is better to be aggressive in getting the Crohn's disease under control before complications such as fistulas and strictures set in. And many GI physicians would agree with this recommendation. But if I can get my patients off milk and tobacco and use agents such as 6-MP and methotrexate, I can generally avoid using Remicade and Humira long term and avoid surgery almost entirely. In fact, I have only one patient on Remicade long term, and none have required Humira. However, I have also given Remicade to three patients to get their Crohn's under control long enough for the 6-MP to kick in. For most of my patients, getting off tobacco and milk products makes their Crohn's much more manageable.

The Three-Step Fiber Therapy Program for Crohn's Disease and Ulcerative Colitis

If you are now ready to try increasing your daily intake of quality fiber, please review the three-step fiber therapy program as outlined in Chapter 3. I also advise starting with Step 1, Week 1 just like everyone else. Remember to go slowly with the program, and don't be surprised if shortly into the program you need to add a laxative. Chapter 3 will help you determine whether and when a laxative is needed. Please don't just rush into a high-fiber diet willy-nilly, as it will probably make you worse rather than better. You know you have an ornery gut, with which you have been living for months, if not years. Please follow the medically tested program outlined in Chapter 3. Chapter 7 adds a few nuances peculiar to IBS patients, and I encourage you to review that chapter as well.

For more information, visit www.crohnsonline.com and www.ccfa.org.

A PREGNANT WOMAN WITH A BOWEL OBSTRUCTION AND CROHN'S

A few years back, I was asked to render a second opinion on a young woman in the hospital who was in her second trimester of pregnancy with her first child. Ms. G had a long-standing history of Crohn's disease; a few years earlier she'd had surgery for a bowel obstruction, and part of her bowel was removed. When I first saw Ms. G, she had a very distended abdomen because of her pregnancy and all the gas trapped inside her from her bowel obstruction. Severe nausea and vomiting were also present. She was in deep distress.

I remember apologizing, telling her that she would require an NG tube (nasogastric tube—a small tube that is passed through your nose into the stomach—ouch!) to help relieve her bowel obstruction and in order to get her GI tract back on track. During my initial talk with her, I mentioned that milk can often exacerbate Crohn's disease. Her comment? Ms. G said that she didn't need me to tell her that milk made her sick, but all of her doctors kept telling her to drink milk because it was so good for her baby. My response was that if milk made her sick, it was not helping her baby. We also talked about the fact that we could not get rid of her adhesions (scar tissue that had built up because of

Ulcerative Colitis

As I said earlier, ulcerative colitis is limited to the colon, whereas Crohn's disease can involve any part of the gastrointestinal tract. Ulcerative colitis is an inflammatory condition of the inner lining of the colon, whereas Crohn's disease involves the entire wall of the gut. Another unique aspect of ulcerative colitis is that it begins with the rectum and may or may not her prior surgery and Crohn's disease), but I thought that trapped abdominal gas might be contributing to her bowel obstruction.

Ms. G did extremely well once we put the NG tube down into her stomach, and within a couple of days she was able to resume eating regular food. She did not resume drinking milk. The remainder of her pregnancy was uncomplicated, and she delivered a healthy baby. Two years or so later, Ms. G wanted to have a second baby. (If you want to make your GI doctor nervous, tell him that you want to get pregnant again!) I did a colonoscopy and sure enough, we found that her Crohn's disease was still active, but only mildly so. Her second pregnancy was smooth as silk, and without incident, and the only medication that she has taken since my first visit with her in the hospital several years back was Pentasa and a short course of prednisone.

Ms. G is now a faithful proponent of my fiber program and won't let herself get within a mile of milk products. She has not had any further episodes of bowel obstruction, nor has she required surgery. Getting off milk may not entirely solve your Crohn's disease, but it helps make whatever medicines you need more effective.

spread back up the GI tract. If ulcerative colitis involves only the rectum, then it is called ulcerative proctitis, not ulcerative colitis. If it extends farther up the colon, it may involve the left colon or even the entire colon, but no more. A hallmark of ulcerative colitis is bleeding, whereas Crohn's may or may not cause bleeding. Diarrhea and urgency are more typical of ulcerative colitis, whereas pain is more common with Crohn's disease. But once again, there is considerable overlap between

A PROFESSIONAL ATHLETE WITH CROHN'S DISEASE

Many years ago I had a female middle-aged professional athlete who had been unable to play in competition for many years because of her diarrhea and stomach cramps, which she thought were due to her Crohn's disease. Her sport did not allow bathroom breaks during matches, and so for years she had to sit in the bleachers and watch rather than compete. Some ten years earlier, she had also had about a third of her large intestine surgically removed. Ever since, her Crohn's had been inactive based on her colonoscopy results and lab work.

As this was early in my practice, I had not yet grasped that diarrhea could be caused by unrecognized constipation. It was only after many office visits that I was able to put two and two together, and even more years before I could convince her that fiber might be the solution to her woes. After finally giving the fiber program a go, she returned to my office with great news. She had been able to return to professional competition. She told me that thanks to the fiber program, she had returned to the circuit and had recently won a national competition.

ulcerative colitis and Crohn's disease. Like Crohn's disease, ulcerative colitis can cause arthritis, liver problems, and similar skin rashes. With long-standing ulcerative colitis and more extensive involvement of the colon, colon cancer occurs with an increasing frequency. Also like Crohn's disease, in my experience the association of IBS and functional diarrhea with ulcerative colitis is more common than not.

Now I realize that most folks are not in dire straits like Mr. A (see page 212–213). But if the fiber program can help him, more than likely it will help whatever GI issues you are facing.

I should add that for us to get Ms. C's colitis under control (see page 214), she required 6-MP. She was also quite skittish about taking a former chemotherapy agent, but it has made a world of difference for her. The reason why I use 6-MP instead of azathioprine (Imuran) is that there have been reports of a lower incidence of pancreatitis with 6-MP. Also, azathioprine is broken down by the body into 6-MP, so it is not like they are different medications. I also told Ms. C of a medical report from the 1990s that looked at two thousand children with inflammatory bowel disease. The authors believed that 6-MP and azathioprine were safer to use in children than prednisone. Because these medicines have been around for more than thirty years, a generic is available. The main precaution required is frequent blood counts to make certain the patient is not getting too much medicine, as 6-MP and azathioprine can cause anemia and serious low-white-cell-count problems, and infrequently liver damage. So make sure you understand why your doctor thinks they are necessary for you. All medicines have side effects. The question is whether the benefits outweigh them. If you are on one of these medicines, make sure you are getting your blood tests as your doctor advises.

Sooner or later all of my patients with Crohn's disease and ulcerative colitis follow at least some modification of my three-step fiber program. I am now so convinced of the need for the introduction of fiber into their diet that I always discuss its eventual need during my initial evaluation, even if my patients have active colitis at the time of their first office visit. I also tell my patients that I am convinced that fiber may help prevent cancer (see Chapter 10). When my patients understand how my fiber program helps their urgency, seepage, diarrhea,

A MAN WITH SEVERE DIARRHEA
AND COLITIS

Mr. A, a young man in his thirties, came to me for a second opinion. He had poorly controlled severe ulcerative colitis. For more than ten years he had been treated for this disorder by a different GI doctor, and yet he continued having severe diarrhea, passing usually as many as ten to twenty watery stools daily. Not unexpectedly, he had great difficulty even keeping a job. Equally distressing for him was his incontinence, which sometimes occurred as often as once a week. Urgency, stomach cramps, and acid reflux were also major issues for him. He brought in a thick pile of records indicating that his most recent colonoscopy, done a year before, was relatively normal. A stool check for blood in the office was negative. He also reported excess gas, explosive diarrhea, and a foul odor.

Given his history and these test results, I thought it likely that his diarrhea was more closely linked to IBS rather than colitis. When I suggested that perhaps he needed more fiber in his diet, Mr. A looked at me like I was crazy. I mean, can you imagine him sitting across the desk from me, hearing me tell him that he was constipated? But fortunately he was quite sharp mentally, and he listened to my argument: "Why would it smell so bad if it weren't

gas, and cramping issues, they soon become faithful adherents. Some may be on a somewhat lower dose, but they all eventually commit to following some variation of the fiber program.

Remember, when using fiber in managing Crohn's disease and ulcerative colitis. However, it is vitally important to get the inflammation under control first. Then the key is to go slowly with fiber, make sure you start with the right kind of fiber, and not be afraid to take a laxative if you need one. Get your GI doctor on board before you begin. Partial bowel obstruction, which rotting inside of you? And if it is rotting, that means it must be sitting around long enough to do that. You say you are filled with gas. Gas is a waste product, and it is not moving through you. This is constipation, pure and simple. Yes, I know it looks like diarrhea, but excess gas and bad odor, and even loss of control, are telltale signs of constipation to me."

Still finding him resistant, I suggested a scientific experiment. "You've tried everything else," I said. "Let's try a little bit of fiber and see what happens. If you improve, then let's try a little more. If you get worse, call me, and I will try something else." So he tentatively agreed to start a small dose of Citrucel; basically this was Week 1 of Step 1 on the fiber therapy program. Sure enough, his diarrhea began to slow, and his urgency improved as well. He cautiously (and at my urging with each subsequent office visit) began to increase his dose of Citrucel, fearing that almost certainly his diarrhea would get worse once again, when in fact he continued to get better. And as I expected, his reflux, stomach cramps, and abdominal gas all greatly improved or vanished entirely. He also regained complete bowel control.

is occasionally seen with Crohn's disease, is thought to be a relative contraindication to using fiber. Patients with this problem should follow the "low-residue diet." That is, avoid seeds, nuts, raw vegetables such as salads, and the skin of fruits. But I still try to use the fiber program even here. Despite all the research on bowel obstruction, nothing out there, including surgery, can prevent it from coming back.

For more information, visit www.uptodate.com/patients and www.ccfa.org.

A HEAD NURSE WITH COLITIS AND CONSTIPATION

Fifteen years back, a former head nurse asked to see me in the office about her rectal bleeding. Ms. C and I have had a long history of working together, sometimes under difficult circumstances with very sick patients. With her I had coined the motto "There is a method to my madness," and also "We have agreed to disagree." We respected each other's professional abilities, but over the years we had also disagreed on how to approach certain problems. She was a formidable ally in the hospital.

I was honored to have Ms. C request an office visit. It turned out that she had a long-standing history of constipation, with bathroom stops only a few times a month, in addition to ulcerative colitis that we found at her colonoscopy. Also, Ms. C, like so many others, had initially discounted my "fiber talk," but eventually I connected with her. Once she got on the fiber program, there was no looking back. Now Ms. C makes several bathroom stops a day and follows the instructions for the fiber program to a T. She more than once has told me that people ask her who is a good gastroenterologist in town, and she says, "No, what you want to know is, who is *my* doctor?"

Celiac Sprue

Ten years ago, celiac sprue was considered a rare disorder characterized by major weight loss, severe diarrhea, and the inability to digest and absorb food. During my first fifteen years of private practice, I could recall having made the diagnosis only once, and I had followed only one other patient with this illness.

Today, I am following close to twenty patients with sprue. Based on antibody tests from blood donors, current estimates show that one out of every 150–300 Americans has this illness. This makes sprue among the most common genetic illnesses in the United States. Physicians today should think about this diagnosis when confronted by irritable bowel syndrome (IBS), iron-deficiency anemia, metabolic bone disease (such as osteoporosis), unexplained liver problems, thyroid disease, diabetes, and possibly neuropsychiatric disorders (such as ataxia, depression, anxiety, epilepsy, or even chronic fatigue). This is a major mental adjustment, and I still forget to request as many sprue panels (a blood test to detect sprue) as I should.

Sprue is an allergy to gluten in the diet. Gluten is a protein that is found in wheat, rye, and barley. For some unknown reason, people with sprue develop an intense inflammation in their small intestines when they eat food with gluten in it. The villi of the intestinal lining flatten out or even slough off, making it difficult to absorb essential nutrients, including iron and certain vitamins. If the damage to the small intestine becomes extensive, then it becomes difficult to absorb enough water, protein, fat, and calories, which leads to weight loss and severe diarrhea. The cornerstone of managing sprue is to first consider it. Then confirm the diagnosis with blood tests and/or a small bowel biopsy, and then carefully exclude gluten from the diet. Unfortunately, a diet without gluten is a very restricted diet. But once again, as with Crohn's disease and ulcerative colitis, even though sprue is an allergy to gluten, patients still need to consume adequate dietary fiber and to achieve large bulky stools each day. Only they need fiber that doesn't contain gluten.

A YOUNG MAN WITH DIARRHEA AND AN ANXIETY PROBLEM

In 1990, Mr. D, a young man in his thirties, came into my office to be evaluated for diarrhea. He had had diarrhea since early childhood. His psychiatrist had made the connection between his bowel problems and an underlying anxiety disorder and had treated him for years. This reminded me of what I had learned in a psychology course at Duke: that it was possible to make a rat nervous. First, you teach the rat to press a bar once to get water and twice to get food. He does that for several months, living very happily getting food and water whenever he wants. One day you change the rules. The rat gets shocked if he presses the bar once or twice. Soon you see the rat running around the cage with his hair all frizzed up.

People are like that, too. Can you imagine being a puny kid with diarrhea and stomach cramps like Mr. D and having to live with your illness? Wouldn't you be running around with your hair standing up on end? So, though I never really asked him, I suspect it was the same with Mr. D. Although he had learned to live with his stomach cramps and diarrhea, he decided to seek evaluation of his GI problems one more time. What other reason would he have to come into my office? All of his lab tests were negative as well as his colonoscopy, which perhaps persuaded him to think that it really was all due to his anxiety problem rather than the other way around: that his anxiety was actually due to his illness. I recall having to call Mr. D on the phone to sweet-talk him

Like Mr. D, even when faced with a confirmed diagnosis and carefully following their dietitian's advice, many sprue patients just don't get that much better. I should add that patients who have lived with their sprue for years are generally into coming in "for one last test," an endoscopy so that I could biopsy his small bowel to look for sprue.

Sure enough, the biopsy of his small intestines was positive for sprue. So Mr. D saw a dietitian, and he began doing extensive reading on his own about his illness. I did not see Mr. D for another ten years or so, when he returned to the office complaining of reflux, periodic stomach pain, excess gas with rumbling, and persistent diarrhea with lots of urgency. Although he had put on a few pounds, he was overall not much better off than he was ten years earlier, when we made his sprue diagnosis. He was thinking that somehow he was getting gluten in his diet, even though he was being as careful with his diet as possible. We repeated the endoscopy and this time his small bowel biopsy was normal, with no signs of sprue. So he got my "fiber talk." Mr. D grudgingly started Benefiber (which contains a minute amount of gluten). Only when he pushed up to the maximum dose of Benefiber, combined with apple juice to get his bathroom stops up to speed, did he begin to see major improvement.

Not only have all of his gas and diarrhea problems vanished, but his acid reflux is also subsiding and he no longer needs his twice-daily dose of Nexium. His wife played a vital role in getting his illness under control (I asked her to come along on his office visits), because she could reinforce to him what we had discussed.

more knowledgeable about their illness than dietitians. I recommend fiber to all of my sprue patients, and I have not heard any say that the fiber was working against them. In addition, I recently found out that Konsyl claims to be gluten free.

So don't be shy. Go online or find someone with sprue who lives in your community. Someone may be living right next door, and he or she may be more than happy to share with you the tips of the trade about what foods you can and can't eat. Avoiding foods that contain gluten is only half the battle. Sooner or later, all of my sprue patients understand the importance of a good fiber program for their GI health. Don't resign yourself to having to learn to live with your illness, as Mr. D wanted to do. This is a psychological trap. If you have lived with your illness for years, I understand how easy it becomes to give up hope of ever getting better. Although the fiber program is wonderful for most people and even for those who have been to major medical centers such as the Mayo Clinic and Duke, I'm sorry to say that a handful of people cannot ever seem to get their bathroom habits up to snuff.

Several chain restaurants now cater to patients with sprue, including Carrabba's, Outback, and Chick-fil-A. I'm sure that by the time this book is published, more restaurants will have begun to offer a special nongluten menu. Just keep asking and knocking on doors. Whole Foods, a national grocery store chain, also caters to people with sprue. So living with sprue today is so much easier than only ten years back. Plus you now know about the fiber program, so in that respect you are way ahead of the game. Like Mr. D, you may be blaming your sprue for your problems, when in reality it may just be plain old run-of-the-mill "vitamin F" deficiency problems. Remember the basics: Excess gas and rancid odor signify that you are living with IBS or a variation of IBS that a good fiber program will often be able to fix.

Just as for Crohn's disease and ulcerative colitis, if you have sprue, I suggest beginning with Step 1, Week 1 of the three-step fiber therapy program. I also encourage you to review Chapter 7, which adds a few important caveats about IBS. Most important, don't rush into fiber. Use only fiber types that are gluten free. Benefiber has only trace amounts of gluten, and my patients with sprue have done well with it. Konsyl indicates that it is entirely gluten free, but it is on Step 3 of the program. Also, don't be surprised if you find yourself needing a laxative as your gut adapts to the fiber program.

For more information, visit www.csaceliacs.org and www.celiac.com.

Diverticulosis and Diverticulitis

The best way to think of diverticulosis is as "pockets" on the colon. The colon looks like someone has pushed a ballpoint pen into it from the inside going to the outside, creating small pockets either within the wall of the colon or sometimes continuing on outside it. Sometimes these pockets are large, but to my knowledge, physicians do not make a distinction between large and small diverticula. Most folks don't even know that they have diverticulosis. About 30–40 percent of people have diverticulosis of the colon by age fifty, and this figure rises to 65 percent by age eighty. So it is a common problem, especially as you age. But when it does cause problems, it can cause havoc, including bleeding and pain. Also, know that diverticulosis can occur just about anywhere in your intestines, including your esophagus, stomach, and small intestines. But diverticulosis of the colon is by far and away the most common type and this condition is also the most likely to cause problems.

I will never forget treating one man in his sixties who had lost so much blood that his blood pressure was in the seventies for several hours while he waited in the emergency room for an intensive-care bed. Despite all the blood transfusions and fluids we gave him, he was back in the emergency room several weeks later with another bleeding episode. Needless to say, he ended up in surgery. Bleeding from diverticulosis can be arterial, which explains why sometimes it may be severe.

When diverticulosis pockets become inflamed, it leads to a condition called diverticulitis. With diverticulitis, there is a tear in the wall of the colon, resulting in a small abscess. Sometimes this is a microscopic abscess, but at other times the abscess is much larger and peritonitis can result if the abscess ruptures. Fortunately peritonitis, which can be life-threatening, is uncommon and occurs only when pus spills out into the abdomen. With diverticulitis, patients usually experience continuous and fairly severe pain and fever lasting several days or longer. Although the pain of diverticulitis is usually on the left side down low, sometimes it may occur throughout the whole abdomen or even be limited to the right side, back, or rectal area. Another hallmark of diverticulitis is a change in bowel pattern. Whether the change is toward constipation or diarrhea, your bowels almost always change when you have an attack of diverticulitis. Excess gas and distention are also characteristic symptoms. Don't forget that a change in bowel habits with stomach pain also occurs with IBS, but there is no fever. With diverticulitis the pain is 24/7.

Back in the 1960s, one elderly woman told me there was a heated debate over what actually caused diverticulitis. One group of medical experts believed that eating seeds and nuts brought on attacks, and the other group thought that the disorder was due to an inadequate fiber intake. Although some medical textbooks suggest avoiding seeds and nuts, both Dr. Denis Burkitt and I and others are in the second camp—we believe that diverticulitis is principally due to "vitamin F" deficiency. In fact, at the Mayo Clinic website (www.mayoclinic.com/health/diverticulitis-diet/AN01255), Dr. Michael Picco states that there is no scientific evidence that seeds and nuts cause diverticulitis. In fact, he states that some evidence shows that seeds and nuts as part of a high-fiber diet may actually protect against this disorder. He does qualify this by saying that if you think that seeds and nuts make your diverticulosis worse, by all means avoid them.

Why would a high-fiber diet prevent diverticulitis? Back when I was in medical school taking anatomy class, we looked at a colon that was pockmarked with numerous diverticula all over it, and then we compared it to a healthy colon. The colon with diverticulosis had very thickened walls and was quite stiff. The healthy colon was soft and pliable. A colon that leads an armchair existence in front of the TV set will, over time, begin to have periodic muscle spasms because it never does regular calisthenics and yoga to keep it limber. Air pressure builds up inside the colon sufficient to cause these pockets to form where the walls are weak. Eventually these pockets can rupture, causing bleeding and/or acute diverticulitis.

Another important point is that arthritis medicines such as ibuprofen and naproxen tend to cause more severe attacks of

A MAN FROM CALIFORNIA
WITH DIVERTICULITIS

Mr. J was a sixty-year-old man sent to my office for a colonoscopy. When we discussed his medical history, he told me of his battle with diverticulitis: "Dr. Jones, I had about thirty to forty attacks of diverticulitis during the ten years that I was living in California. Every time I went in to see my doctor, he would give me an antibiotic and tell me to stay away from seeds and nuts. And I did not eat any seeds or nuts that I knew of, but I kept having these recurring attacks of diverticulitis. The antibiotic would do the trick all right, but within a few months of going off them, I would have another attack. Two years ago, I moved back to Fayetteville and saw Dr. Bill Barry. He told me to take Metamucil twice a day. I listened to him, and over the course of the next two years I had only two attacks. And I know that I should have had six to eight attacks, because while I was in California I was averaging three to four attacks each year. And it turns out that both of my attacks came on when I went out of town and forgot to pack my Metamucil." When Mr. J had finished his success story, I looked at him with a grin on my face and told him, "Sounds to me like you need to remember to pack Metamucil for your trips."

diverticulitis. So use them sparingly if you have diverticulosis, and especially if you have had a prior attack. With an acute attack of diverticulitis, physicians instruct their patients to drink only clear liquids until the attack has significantly subsided. Avoid drinking a lot of diet sodas when you are on a clear liquid diet (even if you have diabetes) because artificial sweeteners have a diuretic effect and may cause dehydration. (This is also important if you are being prepped for a colonoscopy.) This is why pilots do not drink diet sodas when they are on a long flight. I also instruct my patients to stop any fiber during this acute phase, and recommend an antibiotic to fight the infection. Once regular food is resumed, I encourage my patients to begin with a small amount of Benefiber, Citrucel, or EZ Fiber and then gradually increase the amount. Recurrent attacks of diverticulitis or diverticular bleeding are considered a surgical indication for removal of the diseased bowel. Your doctor can help you decide whether surgery is indicated.

One of my surgical colleagues, Dr. Paul Nordness, tells the story of a friend who volunteered to serve as a surgeon at a missionary hospital in Africa perhaps ten years ago. There he was asked by a career missionary surgeon to examine a patient who had severe left lower abdominal pain, constipation and fever. When asked for his diagnosis, his friend replied, "Why, he probably has diverticulitis," to which the other surgeon replied, "In the whole African continent you wouldn't be able to find anyone with diverticulitis. Common things being common, this is almost certainly typhoid or possibly tuberculosis!" The point here being that since dietary fiber intake in Africa is much higher and of better quality than the United States, diverticulitis is rare or virtually nonexistent in Africa whereas it is a relatively common ailment here.

My own experience in Africa dates back to 1969, when I joined a church group that visited Zaire (then called the Democratic Republic of the Congo). One day we took a field trip out to the countryside, where we were served cassava for lunch. I always remember the cassava tasting like a baked potato with 2 tablespoons of Metamucil. I could hardly swallow the stuff. Nutritionally, cassava is comparable to the potato but contains twice the fiber content. The point here is that diverticulosis and diverticulitis are rampant in the Western hemisphere yet almost nonexistent in places like rural Africa, and almost certainly this is because our society subsists largely on processed flour and the wrong kind of whole grain breads and pastas (see Chapter 2).

For more information, visit www.uptodate.com/patients.

KEY POINTS TO REMEMBER

- Almost everyone with Crohn's disease, ulcerative colitis, diverticulosis, and even sprue will benefit from the fiber program, but discuss it with your health care provider first.

- Your colitis should be under moderate control before you introduce fiber into your diet.

- Follow the three-step program outlined in Chapter 3. Go slowly!

- Milk products and smoking often exacerbate Crohn's disease.

- Seeds and nuts may help prevent diverticulitis.

- Arthritis medicines such as ibuprofen and naproxen may make attacks of diverticulitis and diverticular bleeding more severe.

CHAPTER 9

Fighting Depression and Fatigue with Fiber

Although it may seem odd to have a chapter on depression and fatigue in a health book on fiber, my patients tell me how much more energetic they feel once the fiber therapy program weaves its magic. In this chapter I also focus on the depression that results from living with an intractable GI illness, one that you just can't shake: excessive gas, pain, nausea, reflux, or whatever greets you every morning when you get up and confront the question of whether you are looking at a good day or a bad day. There is no letting up with your GI illness and its attendant depression, no vacation days. You feel worn down by the daily experience of anxiety, pain, embarrassment from your noisy stomach, and even your inability to eat a nice meal once in a while without worrying about having to run to the bathroom.

Although this form of depression represents only a narrow slice of the U.S. population, its toll on those afflicted is huge, and it is often unrecognized and untreated. This chapter is for those of you who feel that you have lost all hope of ever

A MIDDLE-AGED WOMAN WITH BOWEL CONTROL ISSUES

Mrs. S was a woman in her fifties who came to see me about her IBS. For years, she had been living with stomach cramps that would double her over in pain, periodic severe explosive diarrhea, and lack of bowel control. She had gone to a nationally recognized universal medical center and had undergone scores of tests, including a colonoscopy, to try to determine why she had such severe pain, diarrhea, and loss of bowel control. She was at wit's end.

The last thing that she could remember being told by her specialist was that the only way she would be able to control her diarrhea and attain bowel control would be to have a colostomy done. (A colostomy is a surgical procedure in which the colon is sewn to the abdominal wall.) Well, Mrs. S was mortified that she might need to wear a bag for the rest of her life. And this is not an uncommon reaction for many people. Rather than carrying that old garbage around inside you, now you are keeping it in a bag just outside your body! Mrs. S also reported noxious bathroom odor and excessive gas, all of which told me that she would likely do very well on the fiber program.

Just two months later Mrs. S returned, raving about how her illness had absolutely vanished. She then looked at me squarely

regaining your GI health. You literally feel as if you are trapped by your body with no way out. Incredible as it may seem, some of the tales of woe I hear sound as if the patient is a prisoner of war, with the all-too-common experience of having doctors run test after test, prescribing medication after medication, year after year, but finding nothing to alleviate any of their symptoms, including the resulting depression.

in the eye and said, "You know, two months ago, I stopped at a different filling station to buy gas than where I usually shop. This was right after Hurricane Katrina had caused all that destruction and interrupted the gas supplies to our state. I bumped into an old friend of mine, who just happened to be there also because of the gas crisis, and I suddenly found myself telling her about all of my problems. All she said was, 'You have just got to go see that Dr. Jones in Fayetteville. He will fix you up if anyone can.' You know, I was getting so depressed about my situation that I actually thought about suicide a time or two. Why, I never thought that I could ever live with myself having a colostomy and all. I really didn't think I could do that."

Thinking back to my conversation that afternoon with Mrs. S, I could not help but notice how different she looked from her initial visit two months earlier. I had never suspected her of being suicidal, but I did recall the desperation in her face when we first talked about her problems. Here was a woman in her fifties who had been trapped by her body. And even if she wore diapers, they would not solve the odor and noise problem. She had seen scads of doctors, and until her visit to my office, no one had been able to help her. As Mrs. S left the exam room, you could almost see her floating down the hall, so transformed was her outlook on life.

People with reactive depression often experience feelings of worthlessness, sleep disorders, loss of appetite, weight loss, and even thoughts about death and suicide. Naturally, their marriages suffer, as do relationships with their children and close friends. My intent in this chapter is to clarify for you how common these forms of reactive depression and chronic fatigue are, and yet how treatable.

A FORMER GANG MEMBER WITH SEVERE PAIN AND WEIGHT LOSS

One day a few years back when I was on hospital call for our GI specialty group, I was asked to see a man with severe stomach pain and constipation. Mr. K, thirty years old, had once been a gang member in another state and had spent time in prison. A few years back, he had developed an AIDS-like illness as well as a condition called *colonic pseudo-obstruction*, for which I was consulted. In colonic pseudo-obstruction, the colon basically shuts down. Everything the person eats that the body cannot digest stays trapped inside the gut.

In *Merriam-Webster's Collegiate Dictionary*, Eleventh Edition, *pseudo* is defined as "being apparently rather than actually as stated." This means that on the X-ray studies, the colon only looked as if it were blocked, rather than having an actual obstruction. With this illness, the colon is tremendously enlarged with liters of trapped gas inside. The abdomen is hugely distended, and people with this problem often look like pregnant women on the cusp of delivery. Mr. K had seen at least one gastroenterologist at a major teaching medical center, where he'd had a colonoscopy and an endoscopy as well as all sorts of X-ray studies. He was given a slew of different medications in an attempt to help his GI tract, but all to naught. He had been in and out of hospitals for the preceding eighteen months, and he finally decided to move back to the Fayetteville area, because it was home for him. Basically, his team had decided that his colonic pseudo-obstruction was related to either his AIDS or the medications he was taking for it. They concluded that nothing more could be done to help him.

When I went to see Mr. K, he was in isolation because he was thought to possibly have tuberculosis. Despite having lost more than fifty pounds, he was still a big man with a huge frame, and I clearly remember feeling his hostility as I walked into his room. When I sat down, he just glared at me. I'm sure I looked like all the other doctors before who had been unable to help. All they did was run all kinds of tests and give him all sorts of pills, and here he was, just the same as always if not worse. His responses to my questions were hollow and just a few words at most. He seemed to only half-listen to my questions.

Yes, he was constipated. Yes, he had tried Metamucil, Citrucel, magnesium citrate, Zelnorm, lactulose, enemas, MiraLax, and all sorts of laxative pills. Nothing other than enemas had worked for him, but they helped only for a day or so at most. Then everything came back again. Not that I had expected otherwise. He had severe, continuous stomach pain and, as I had expected, his abdomen was tightly distended because of all the gas that was trapped inside. I went back to my office and studied his files. All his lab studies and exams were negative. I next looked at Mr. K's X-rays, including his CT scan, with the only remarkable finding being a hugely dilated colon filled with gas and stool.

So I went back upstairs and visited once again with Mr. K. I told him I was not certain I could help, but I thought that just possibly I could. I distinctly remember explaining to Mr. K the idea of the colon being like a railroad car and how it takes thirty men to get it rolling down the tracks. But once that old heavy railroad car gets rolling along at a good clip, old-timers said it takes only two men to keep it moving. Because his colon did not have an actual blockage, I told him we were going to have to use thirty men to get his colon moving again. From what he told me, it looked like the thirty men were going to be the old, trusty tap-water enema and that gallon

(continued)

jug of NuLytely he'd had to drink to get his colonoscopy done; those were the only tricks left in my doctor's bag. I didn't have anything else to offer, but I suggested that we try the water enemas as often as twice a day; once we got results, we would have him start drinking 2 or 3 quarts of NuLytely each day. Then once we got his old railroad car moving down the tracks, we could start introducing a small amount of high-quality fiber twice a day into his system. Eventually I hoped that we would be able to switch him over to Milk of Magnesia or citrate of magnesia, instead of drinking several quarts of NuLytely every day. That was the game plan, and I laid it all out in lurid detail. I thought it was important that he could see where we were headed, and not just enemas for the rest of his life.

You could see Mr. K looking me up and down, trying to decide whether I was sincere and whether going through the embarrassment of an enema as often as twice a day was worth the effort. Oh, he had had enemas before, but nobody had ever recommended that he take them daily, much less twice a day. He also worried that the enemas might make his colon even worse. "Can't you get dependent on those things?" he asked. I reassured him that hopefully, what we were going to do would make his colon stronger, not weaker. I told him about some of the people who had tried the program in past years and how it had helped them. I also reminded him that he had tried everything else. What the heck—we could try this for a week or so and see if we could get his bowels moving, and just maybe we could get him eating again. So Mr. K decided to give it a try, and he began with twice-daily warm-water enemas plus drinking several quarts of

Perhaps you have even taken an antidepressant medication, but without much help. This is probably because the GI illness that caused your problems in the first place was never successfully managed. In essence, trying to treat reactive depression

NuLytely every day. I also got some raised eyebrows from the nurses who had to give him all those enemas.

After the first week, Mr. K was discharged from the hospital feeling better, especially because he was also able to resume eating without severe pain and gas. In follow-up visits to my office, he often brought his father. He was making good progress with his bowels, not needing the enemas as often as before and, most important, not having to go back to the hospital. In fact, he found that he could use an enema to stop his stomach from hurting after he ate. He was definitely eating better, and best of all, his weight was up. Mr. K then started taking the Benefiber just as I had asked—going slowly and taking a little more every week. About a year after my first visit with him in the hospital, Mr. K walked into my office and sat down with a huge grin on his face. He told me that he had stopped his enemas completely several months earlier, but he still needed an occasional Milk of Magnesia to keep his bowels on track, in addition to the Metamucil and oatmeal that he was now taking.

He then told me that he had gone back to church and was talking with the youth about steering clear of drugs and gangs. What a stark contrast in his demeanor from my first visit with him only twelve months earlier! He then looked at me and told me that when I had first walked in to see him only a year earlier, he knew his back was to the wall and at the time, suicide seemed like it was his only way out of his situation. No question about it. Here was a man transformed by the fiber program—changing from a demeanor of anger and depression only a year earlier to a man now radiating warmth, faith, and good cheer.

under these circumstances is like taking Tylenol for pneumonia. Your temperature may be down, but you won't feel much better until your pneumonia is being controlled with the right antibiotic. I often know how my patients are doing in the bathroom just by walking into the exam room. A former office nurse once even commented, "Your IBS patients are often beaming when they come into your office. What a contrast from other offices where I have worked, where the IBS patients generally walk in with sad faces, sometimes even hunched over."

In my mind, the preceding two patients (see pages 226–231) had experienced a reactive depression to their catastrophic IBS-like illnesses, as evidenced by their contemplations of suicide and death. Facing illness day after day, with no hope of getting better, can be devastating to the psyche. Here, solving their severe IBS-like illness riddle was central to overcoming their depression. But the rapidity of the resolution of their depressive complaints without medication was also quite remarkable.

Fighting Fatigue

My mother's bathroom habits are a running joke in the family. I guess you could even say that I was "home-schooled" by my mother in the sense that her constipation problems have been an issue for her as far back as I could remember! Nothing like having roots for a book like this! Her entire day revolved around whether she was successful in the bathroom. At eighty-nine she still will not leave the house without first doing what needs to be done in the bathroom. Out-of-town trips for my parents always were scheduled after eleven A.M. for this reason. My businessman father just learned to live with her problem, as frustrating as it was for him, as there was nothing he could do about it if he wanted her to travel with him. Years ago, I did not understand why my mother was this way, but now that I'm older and wiser, the matter is no longer a subject of amusement, but rather more a statement on life in general. Bowel habits are critical to many folks, and this is especially true as one ages.

In the old days, before modern corrective surgery had arrived, if a kid grew up with a club foot and nothing was ever done about it, he or she went through life knowing running as more of a hop and skip than actual running like the wind. The same is true of bathroom habits. If you have always had poor bathroom stops with small rancid stools and gas, from your perspective that is normal—just like those young women who felt fine even though they were in the bathroom to move their bowels only once a month. The sluggishness and fatigue creeps in ever so slowly. Often you attribute these feelings to the aging process; you start feeling tired as soon as you get up in the morning.

Twenty years ago a radiology friend of mine suddenly lost his voice. While waiting for the test results, he became so frightened at the thought that he might have laryngeal cancer that he stopped his two-pack-a-day smoking habit cold turkey. Now he comments on how much better he feels since he stopped smoking. He had attributed his sluggishness and general malaise to getting older, not realizing how much his smoking actually affected his body. Only once he had quit did he realize the impact heavy smoking was having on his energy level. It was like night and day.

So it can be for those of you who discover what normal bowel habits were intended to be. It is like learning to breathe—something that folks only a century ago took for granted. People back then knew how important it was to stay on top of your bowels, and to take a laxative if they were not having good results. Today it is the other way around. Only when they are having major issues with constipation does anyone consider reaching for a laxative. This is a mistake because constipation is much easier to control when it is just getting started than days or weeks later. And then people sell themselves short by shooting for a small stool once or twice a day when what they really need are several excellent bathroom stops daily.

But remember also that even several stools every day does not mean you are out of the woods. Foul odor is the red flag. That is why colonic irrigation is so popular among the elderly. If you have spent time on the interstate highways, especially the ones en route to Florida, I'm sure that you have seen those giant billboards advertising colonics. Advertising on billboards is expensive, so you know there must be a lot of money spent on the business. But frankly, getting your colon irrigated must be a bit embarrassing, and it just isn't natural to have a tube stuck up your rear end on a regular basis to make you feel better. At least when we do a colonoscopy, we give you a strong sedative and a narcotic, so that most folks are not even aware of their exam.

Those who give colonics know that they are making their patients feel better. But within the next few days, the problem of sluggishness and fatigue is right back because everything is just sitting there putrefying inside you all over again. Trust me. When you have a colonic irrigation, that garbage bag of leftovers leaves the room for a day, but then it sneaks right back inside. Right idea, wrong approach. You need to get all of those undigested leftovers out of your system as expeditiously as possible, and within twenty-four hours, not several days. And by your own effort, not by having someone else do it for you. For

A WOMAN WITH SEVERE ARTHRITIS
WHO WAVED HER CANE

Mrs. A, a petite woman in her seventies, has been a patient of mine for many years. She is a stoic woman who lives with severe degenerative arthritis. She has a long-standing history of IBS, diarrhea predominant, which was especially troublesome whenever she traveled out of town. Mrs. A did quite well with her own modified version of the fiber program for many years, having never quite accepted the goal I advised because she was so petite in her build. Last summer, Mrs. A had a severe flare-up of her arthritic back pain, and simultaneously her old IBS reared its ugly head once more. She was hospitalized twice in the subsequent six months for severe attacks of stomach pain and gas. She felt so miserable that she became a shut-in, not even going to see the doctor unless she absolutely had to. During the last time she was in the hospital, I connected with her. I told her point blank that either she should learn to live with her intestinal problems or else she should carefully follow the fiber therapy program. I gave her the same fiber instruction sheets as before. This time, her son and daughter-in-law, who lived across the street, made certain that she stayed on the program. One day recently, she spotted me at a social function and walked up with a great big smile on her face. What really caught my eye was how she was waving her cane as she ambled over to chat. That waving of her cane up in the air was a nonverbal cue as to how much more energy she was feeling, not to mention that she was now well enough to get out of her house and socialize. Her comment: "I had locked myself up in the house these past six months because I did not feel well enough to do anything. I was too miserable even to go see the doctor!"

I HAVE A GREAT BACK AND A LOUSY NECK

For years I have told people I had one of the best backs in the world. You hear about bad backs everywhere, but no one talks about having a great back. You see, my back talks to me all the time. Twenty-five years ago my back put up such a ruckus that I had to drop out of work for a few days, and back then I did what most folks did: I took a bunch of medicine and went to bed. But I soon pulled out an orthopedics book and began doing exercises, at first three and four times daily, but as the years passed I needed to do those exercises only once or twice daily. For twenty years I did really well, with my back talking to me if I ever got slack about the program. But five years ago, my back was no longer satisfied, and it started making a lot more noise, so I went and saw a local chiropractor. He fixed me up, but the problem came back again a few months later.

Having seen all of the problems that pain and arthritis pills can cause, I steered clear of them and started yoga and began seeing another chiropractor. It turns out that gastroenterologists frequently have musculoskeletal issues because of the nature of our work. When we are scoping, we are almost always turned the same way and tilted a little, and so various musculoskeletal injuries are common in our profession, particularly as we age. Now although I have a great back that talks to me all the time, my neck is a lousy communicator. Five years ago, boom! It happened. No warning at all. All of a sudden, I popped a disc in my neck. Nothing helped. I could hardly walk, so within two or three weeks, I had surgery. For some people their GI tracts are much like my back, and yet for other people they are like my neck. For those who are like my back, their guts like to complain a lot. But not everyone's guts complain so noisily and they are like my neck. Instead these folks have no warning that there may be a problem just around the next bend in the road.

A WOMAN WITH A CHIP ON HER SHOULDER

Mrs. E and I sat down in the exam room to discuss her liver problems, rehashing the uncertain issues and agreeing on a plan of management. With that out of the way, I asked her about her bowel habits and how her energy level was doing, well knowing about her lifelong battle with constipation. She lit up immediately. "All my life, the only times I ever went to the bathroom were during my menstrual cycle; this was at most a few times a month, and otherwise I did not go at all. Because I felt fine, I thought my bowel pattern was healthy. In fact, I took my children to see the pediatrician because I thought something must be wrong, because they were going every day. I had never done that in my whole life. The doctor told me that going to the bathroom every day was normal for some people. Boy, was I ever surprised. I really thought my kids might be sick or something."

She went on. "Yes, I am making good progress with the fiber program, and my energy level is indeed much better. But that is not the half of it, as far as I am concerned. The most profound change is that I am so much more cheerful. Even my family has noticed. My husband has now gotten interested in the success of my bathroom program. Why, he has several times called me at work to say that he noticed that I was getting low on my laxative supply and wanted to know if he could pick up a few bottles from the store."

I looked at Mrs. E and said, "Thinking back, when you first came to see me, I thought something was wrong. Because you work in an attorney's office, I wondered if perhaps you might be looking for a reason to sue. I used to think you had a chip on your shoulder or something. I didn't know what it was, but I always had this uneasy feeling around you whenever you came for a visit." Mrs. E replied, "That's true. Back then, I really did have a chip on my shoulder! People that I have not seen in years have noticed how much I have changed."

this reason, the colonic irrigation will never be able to match the results of a good fiber program—unless, of course, you decide to have your irrigation done twice daily for the rest of your life! I guess somebody may be doing that, but most folks just don't have the dollars or time to spend on this.

When you embrace the fiber program (and adding a laxative if necessary to get your bathroom stops up to speed), you will never look back, realizing how much better you feel. That is why people in their seventies and eighties today often can remember their parents or grandparents telling them to take a laxative once a week or so, because their parents (and grandparents) had grown up on a diet of high-quality fiber and clearly knew the difference between subpar bathroom results and good results and how this affected their sense of general well-being.

Many doctors think their patients with IBS are just wimps or grouches, when in reality, I suspect they are a lot tougher in dealing with their pain than their doctor will ever be. Never one to complain, they go through life merrily on their way carrying their garbage bag of leftovers putrefying inside of them year in and year out. But without a moment's notice, all of sudden it happens. Boom!

It may be an attack of diverticulitis, a gallbladder attack, or a bad bout with reflux that makes them go to the emergency room to get their heart checked out—or it may be something subtle, such as loss of appetite and even gradual weight loss. Chronic fatigue and sluggishness may not always be caused by constipation, but I suspect it is much more common than generally recognized.

What the heck, the fiber program is good for your health. Why not give it a spin? Recently, while we were setting up for a colonoscopy, I chatted with one of my patients about her progress with the fiber program. One of the GI nurses suddenly chimed in and said, "Boy, I sure can tell when I get sidetracked and get off Dr. Jones's program. Why, I just feel dead at the end of the day. I have no energy; I'm just miserable. What a difference in how I feel when I stay on top of my bowels. That's why I sent my whole family to see Dr. Jones, because I've seen what a difference his fiber program has made in my life."

Everybody knows that if their bowels move every day, they feel much better than if they moved their bowels only a few times a week or less often. Is it that far of a stretch to understand that making bathroom stops several times a day, especially if stools are large and soft with minimal odor, will give you even more zip to your gait? Remember that Dr. Denis Burkitt said that the United States and Great Britain are constipated nations. We agree that this widely prevalent disorder is wreaking untold havoc on the United States, much like the silent killers of tobacco and hypertension. It may be hard to believe but both Dr. Burkitt and I are convinced that poor bowel habits are as devastating to a person's health as tobacco, hypertension, and obesity.

KEY POINTS TO REMEMBER

- Reactive depression caused by GI illnesses such as IBS may be devastating to a person's psyche and yet sometimes is easily managed by controlling the underlying GI disorder.

- You wouldn't carry a bag of rotting garbage slung over your back all day long, so why do you let the stuff sit inside you all day? Why should you be surprised that some days you have no energy and even feel sad and blue?

- Just as chain smokers don't recognize that their fatigue and malaise are tobacco related, people often don't realize how much of a problem their constipation is.

CHAPTER 10

Cancer, Alzheimer's Disease, and the High-Fiber Diet

Ever held a baby in your arms? You cannot help but be struck by the luster of the baby's skin and pristine appearance. Now gaze at an elderly octogenarian ambling slowly on a sidewalk, so stiff rather than limber like that baby. And it is not just all those years of being out in the sunlight that makes octogenarians look old; even their internal organs and their reflexes are not the same. Is there any way to delay the aging process? Could our bodies really be like an aquarium? Could doing a better job keeping our internal filters clear make a difference? More to the point, are cancer and Alzheimer's disease inevitable conditions that most of us must face as we age? If we cannot change our genes, can we delay the onset of these illnesses?

I believe that the answer to this last question is a resounding "Yes!" My premise is that a good-quality fiber program has a double-pronged attack for protecting your body. The first is moving all those leftovers out of your body in a timely manner, thereby interrupting the putrefaction process that would otherwise occur. You don't want to have food rotting inside you. But a second and probably equally important benefit of a high-quality fiber program is that it scrubs your bile, helping your liver do its job. The liver and kidneys are the mainstays of ridding your body of any accumulated toxins and waste. In this chapter my theories about the relationship between constipation and Alzheimer's disease and cancer are purely speculative, based on a series of seemingly isolated observations. Most scientists would not be impressed with such a methodology. But the possibility that current scientific research on cancer and Alzheimer's disease could be turned upside down and the incidence and prevalence of these dreaded diseases could be dramatically reduced with a simple high-fiber diet cannot be just dismissed out of hand. And although this is only a theory, I expect that one day science will have to either prove or disprove it.

A lecture I attended at Duke University Medical School in the early 1970s flashed in front of me. The professor had shown slides illustrating the steadily rising incidence of almost all types of cancer in the United States. He next showed slides on cancer mortality among Mormons as being much lower than the U.S. population as a whole. No one knew why Mormons had such low rates of cancer, he said. Although Mormons don't drink coffee or tea, careful epidemiological studies had shown that this was not the reason. "No one can explain their low incidence of cancer," he concluded.

I had noticed something similarly inexplicable in Bolivia, where I have worked each year at the Alfonso Gumucio Reyes Hospital in concert with Consejo de Salud Rural Andino (CSRA). (CSRA is a health care project based in Bolivia that

A MORMON WITH IBS

One December afternoon in 1995, Mrs. B, a woman in her midthirties, came into my office complaining of stomach pain and altered bowel habits consistent with a diagnosis of irritable bowel syndrome (IBS). After taking her medical history and giving her a physical exam, I began talking to her about fiber and how her problem could be helped. To my surprise, Mrs. B suddenly began chuckling. She said, "You just told me I'm not a good person." I looked at her quizzically, and she repeated her comment. "You just told me I'm not a good person."

Mrs. B then went on to explain that she was Mormon. She said that the Mormon Bible tells its followers to grind their wheat at home and to avoid processed, store-bought flour and baked wheat products. She told me she had a grinder and two bags of wheat at home, but she had been just too busy to grind it into flour, much less bake it into bread. She added, "You just intimated that if I had been a more faithful Mormon, I would not have gotten sick in the first place."

is a sister organization of Curamericas Global, Inc., of which I am the current board chair.) When I first arrived in Montero in November 1987, one of the remarks I often heard was, "We just don't have any cancer here in Bolivia. It must be the water or something." Indeed, during my first six years working in Bolivia, spending two weeks each year and seeing about 150 patients during each trip, I encountered only one woman in her eighties who had pancreatic cancer. I also seldom found any polyps at colonoscopy.

Then suddenly, in June 1995, only a few months before my office visit with Mrs. B, the young Mormon woman with IBS,

I saw six patients with cancer at the Montero hospital. By my twelfth trip to Bolivia in 2000, I had encountered an additional fourteen cancer patients, bringing the total to twenty. Though this sample was clearly limited, the cancer incidence in this region of Bolivia appeared to have exploded roughly twenty-fold. And the cancer locations varied extensively, arising in such places as the pelvis, colon, stomach, esophagus, and breast. At the conclusion of one recent trip, Dr. Joel Horowitz, a cancer surgeon, commented, "I can't believe how much cancer I saw here!" And last summer, I saw a forty-year-old woman with half of her stomach filled with cancerous tumors.

What happened? Why did cancer suddenly appear in Bolivia in the mid-1990s? Although patients traveled hundreds of miles from all across the country, most of the people I saw lived within a hundred miles of Montero, where I work. On my return visit to Bolivia in 1996, thinking over what my Mormon patient had said, I decided to speak with the late Walt Henry and his wife, Susie, both of whom had worked as missionaries to Bolivia since the early 1960s. I also wanted to see what Dr. Dardo Chávez, a native physician and personal friend who is also the project director of CSRA, made of the rise in cancer cases. I was especially interested in what they could tell me about dietary changes they had witnessed.

Walt, Susie, and Dardo all told me that processed white flour first became widely prevalent in the Montero/Santa Cruz area of Bolivia sometime around the 1960s. I have subsequently confirmed this with a number of other physicians in Bolivia.

Any bona fide epidemiologists would be shaking their heads right now, well recognizing that the preceding anecdotes only show *association* rather than proving *causality*. Only scientific methodology and statistics can support my theorizing, and both are very exacting. To support a link between the presence of a bacteria and an illness, according to Koch's postulates, (1) the bacteria first must be isolated from a diseased animal; (2) next, the bacteria must be grown in culture in a lab; (3) these bacteria grown in culture must then be injected into a different animal, with subsequent appearance of the same illness; and finally, (4) the same strain of bacteria as was originally found in the diseased animal back in step 1 must be isolated and identified.

For instance, Crohn's disease has long been suspected as being caused by a bacterial infection, but to date, Koch's postulates have not been fully met. So the proposed bacterial cause of Crohn's disease has not enjoyed much credibility among physicians for this reason. This is real science, and the reader should understand that what this chapter offers is pure speculation.

However, I hope that this chapter will reopen the question of *autointoxication*, which was first proposed by Elie Metchnikoff, a Russian biologist. Metchnikoff shared the Nobel Prize for his work in immunology in 1908. Metchnikoff proposed that the body absorbs decomposing toxic waste products in the colon, which leads to various degenerative illnesses as one ages. In the early part of the twentieth century, Dr. J. H. Kellogg at the Battle Creek Sanitarium in Michigan supported Metchnikoff's theory, and Kellogg himself also felt that passing several stools daily was one of the keys to general good health. However, with his breakfast cereals, Kellogg did have a vested financial interest in his recommendations. So I am not really proposing a new theory, just resurrecting an old one.

In a recent informal conversation with the late Dr. Paul

Killenberg, former professor of medicine at Duke in the department of gastroenterology, he commented that sunspot activity or expanding holes in the ozone layer of Earth's atmosphere may also be linked with the global spike in cancer rates that we have witnessed, but that doesn't mean that this phenomenon definitively caused the spike. I had to agree with Dr. Killenberg's comments. However, I believe that several other observations and insights merit our attention and perhaps indirectly strengthen this autointoxication theory as proposed by Metchnikoff a century ago.

What Is Cancer?

Almost everybody knows that cancer often spreads before it can be surgically removed, ultimately leading to death if not caught in its earliest stages. However, most folks really don't know what cancer is and why it does what it does. To a physician or scientist, *cancer* means an abnormal clustering of cells that, if unchecked, will tend to continue expanding into the surrounding tissues and often will spread to other parts of the body. As with everything else in medicine, there are exceptions to this rule. For example, leukemia (and a few other cancers) do not show these cell clusters.

Some experts have described cancer cells as being immortal. This means that cancer cells don't generally die, as do most other cells in the body, and more important, they just keep dividing, or rather replicating. During the first two decades of your life, your arms, legs, and spine grow to a certain distance and then stop, but not so for cancer cells. They just keep dividing and piling up on top of one another, and this process goes on unchecked indefinitely. This uncontrolled growth of cancer cells eventually leads to local invasion of whatever tissue or organ is adjacent. If a blood vessel or lymphatic vessel is nearby, a few cancer cells often catch a ride to distant tissue sites and settle down to grow in the liver, bone, lung, or even brain, but they can grow practically anywhere.

Some cancers have been shown to be caused by viruses, such as Burkitt's lymphoma, which is caused by the Epstein-Barr virus. Other cancers are clearly caused by carcinogens (chemicals that cause cancer). Working in a cobalt mine years ago meant that you would probably die of lung cancer. Tar in cigarettes is thought to cause lung cancer, and smoked foods are believed to cause stomach cancer. Genes also clearly play a role. As an example, experts believe that 5 percent of colon cancers are caused by genes received from the patient's parents. If you have the HNPCC (hereditary nonpolyposis colorectal cancer) gene, then you have a 70–90 percent chance of developing colorectal cancer if you live long enough. However, 95 percent of patients with colorectal cancer do not have any known family history of the disease. So, even if your family history is negative for colon cancer, you should still consider having a screening exam for this illness. If you wait until you are having symptoms such as rectal bleeding or change in bowel habits, then there is only perhaps a 50 percent chance that your surgeon will be able to remove your cancer completely. A family history is also important for most other cancers. For instance 15–20 percent of women who develop breast cancer have a positive family history. Further, individual family trees of people with HNPCC show that the grandparents typically developed their cancer in their sixties or seventies, whereas their grandchildren developed their cancer in their thirties and forties—again suggesting that even when genetics are thought to play a key role in cancer development, some environmental factor is probably also at work.

Although there is really nothing concrete here, all of these observations are interesting when viewed in the light of the autointoxication theory advocated by Metchnikoff. So I began trying to determine, in a purely informal and ad hoc way, whether there was any correlation between the switch from whole wheat and bran to processed flour and the spike in cancer cases in America.

The Egyptians were thought to have baked yeast bread as early as 2600 B.C. However, for centuries, most people ate whole-wheat or whole-grain bread. Not until the late 1800s was machinery invented that allowed the mass production of milled white flour. Inexpensive processed white-flour bread probably became widely available around 1900. Digging further, I found that Nabisco was founded in 1898 by the merger of three baking companies with 114 bakeries under their management. Barnum's Animal Crackers were introduced in 1902; Lorna Doone and Oreo cookies were released in 1912. The Kellogg Company was founded in 1906 to mass market its hugely successful flagship product, Corn Flakes. Rice Krispies were first marketed in 1928. General Mills debuted Kix Cereal in 1937 and Cheerioats (now called Cheerios) in 1941. So although processed flour was available in the United States since the mid- to late 1800s, only during the beginning of the twentieth century did the consumption of popular low-fiber cereals, white breads, and snacks become widespread. During World War II,

Great Britain decided that white-flour products were a luxury the country could not afford, so the government mandated that all wheat products be whole grain and unprocessed. This reinforces the idea that white flour was considered a luxury during the early part of the twentieth century, when the United States was predominantly a rural/agricultural nation. Keeping this timeline in mind, I next looked at what I could find out about the widespread arrival of cancer in the United States.

For many years I have been under the impression that cancer became widely prevalent in the United States by the 1950s. In fact, one woman recalls being told that her mother was the first person to ever be diagnosed with cancer in High Point, North Carolina, during the 1950s. Because High Point is only a stone's throw from the city of Greensboro, lack of available medical evaluation cannot explain this. Some may argue that the widespread arrival of cancer in the United States in the twentieth century can be explained equally well by an improvement in diagnosis or greater access to health care, because after World War II, almost certainly more doctors were available to serve more people, since many of the military physicians returned to civilian careers at the conclusion of the war. As an example, many epidemiologists explain the explosion in autism diagnosis with the arrival of the field of child psychology. However, as we shall see, the rise of cancer in the United States occurred well before World War II. While reviewing the U.S. National Center for Health Statistics website, I found reams of data dating back to 1900.

Admittedly we should be cautious interpreting health data derived a century ago. Modern medicine was only in its infancy at that time, and the tools available to physicians to determine cause of death were crude by contemporary standards. But evidence shows that recorded death statistics are reasonably reliable (more about this later in the chapter). In fact, the ancient world was quite familiar with cancer. The first recorded descriptions of cancer date as far back as 1500 B.C. (3,500 years ago!), and the first case of mastectomy for breast cancer was reported by the Roman medical writer Celsus almost 2,000 years ago! An old pathology textbook—James Ewing's *Neoplastic Diseases*, published by W. B. Saunders in 1919—describes in surprisingly accurate detail the pathologies of common cancers. I was also surprised to learn that autopsies were performed by the tens of thousands during the nineteenth century.

I found some eye-catching statistics. In 1900, the United States had a population of 76 million, and yet barely 12,000 cancer deaths were recorded that year; cancer represented only 3.7 percent of the total reported cause of death. By 1950, the U.S. population had nearly doubled. In that year, 210,000 deaths were attributed to cancer, accounting for 14.5 percent of all deaths. By 2000 the population had nearly doubled again to 281 million, and with 561,000 cancer deaths—23.3 percent of all deaths. In essence, total cancer deaths had climbed well over *sixteenfold* from 1900 to 1950, yet the U.S. population had only doubled in as many years. However, from 1950 to 2000, total cancer deaths again increased, but by less than a factor of threefold, when the U.S. population once again had doubled.

In addition, most of this further increase in cancer deaths in the latter part of the twentieth century was due to lung cancer (discussed shortly). Another way to put this is that in 1900 there were 17 cancer deaths annually for every 100,000 people. By 1950, this figure had risen to 140 cancer deaths for every 100,000 population, or a more than an eightfold increase. By the year 2000, there were almost 200 cancer deaths annually for every 100,000 people in the United States, and much of this increase was largely due to the rapid rise in lung cancer, with lung cancer deaths being only 14 per 100,000 population in 1950, and rising to 59 per 100,000 in 1995.

Taking lung cancer mortality figures out of the data analysis, I noted only a marginal increase in cancer mortality from 1950 to 2000, despite the widespread arrival of preservatives and insecticides in the middle of the twentieth century. It appears that cancer had become well entrenched in the United States by 1950, and the continued increase in cancer mortality beyond 1950 was largely due to the arrival of lung cancer. Smoking was mass-marketed during both World Wars, with packs of cigarettes included in soldier ration packs. Mass production of rolled cigarettes began in the late 1800s.

These cancer figures are more interesting when we consider that the widespread arrival of processed white flour came only a few decades ahead of cancer. There is a difference, however, between the United States and Bolivia. The rise of cancer in the Montero/Santa Cruz area was even more dramatic than what occurred in the United States. I suspect that this is partly because the United States is much larger and has a more heterogeneous population than Bolivia. Research also has demonstrated that the smaller the population studied, the more frequent are larger variations from the norm. However, I remain struck by the fact that people in the United States recall the arrival of cancer in their communities, and the U.S. National Center for Health Statistics website corroborates their observations.

U.S. Cancer Mortality (in Thousands) by Age Group When Lung Cancer Is Excluded

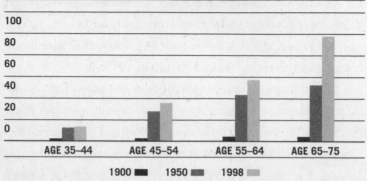

1900 ■   1950 ■   1998 ▨

Some will argue that because cancer is an illness of the aged, and because people lived longer in the latter part of the twentieth century, cancer would thus be expected to be more prevalent than a hundred years ago. Indeed, life expectancy was 47.3 years in 1900, 68.2 years in 1950, and 77 years in 2000. But if we look at individual age groups, we find that cancer deaths increased between *tenfold and twentyfold* across the board (see the accompanying bar graph) between 1900 and 1950. There was a further increase in cancer deaths after 1950, but the most pronounced changes occurred before 1950. As an example, for people ages 55–64, there was an almost sixteenfold increase in cancer deaths between 1900 and 1950; of total deaths for this age group, the proportion of those attributed to cancer rose from 9.7 per 100,000 population to 20.5 per 100,000 population. I am uncertain why cancer mortality continued to rise rapidly for the 65–74 age group between 1950 and 1998, but I suspect that this may be due to a combination of factors, but most likely due to the rising risk of lung cancer in smokers as they age. Looking at breast cancer, we find that in the United States there were 5.6 deaths per 100,000 population in 1914, 12.5 deaths per 100,000 population in 1950, and only a slight rise to 16.9 deaths per 100,000 population in 1985.

No matter how you look at the death statistics, they generally support the idea that cancer became well established in the United States by 1950, and yet it was relatively uncommon only five decades earlier.

So what else happened between 1900 and 1950? The first crop duster airplanes for spraying crops with insecticide arrived sometime in the 1920s. However, because of the Depression and its associated economic crisis, almost certainly the widespread use of crop-dusting airplanes did not occur until after World War II, when the United States was finally on its way to economic recovery. Furthermore, effective organic insecticides did not arrive until the 1940s. For instance, DDT was first recognized to be useful as an effective insecticide in 1939. Thus, the dramatic rise in cancer deaths during the first five decades of the twentieth century probably cannot be ascribed to the widespread use of insecticides.

It is more difficult to get a handle on food preservatives because food additives have been used since the beginning of recorded history. They include alcohol, salt, sugar, and vinegar (natural preservatives), antioxidants (BHA and BHT), antimicrobial products (sodium nitrate, sodium nitrite, sulfites, EDTA, calcium proprionate, etc.) and not to mention smoked foods. I am not aware of any compelling evidence that implicates food preservatives and additives as causing cancer, with the primary exception being smoked foods and stomach cancer. If any such evidence existed, then almost certainly there would be a public outcry, similar to the outcry against DDT that led to its ban from the U.S. market in 1972.

"Doctors didn't know what cancer was back then, or else they couldn't diagnose it because the medical technology was so primitive." I have heard this comment by skeptical patients many times. My response has been, "Yes, a small lump in a woman's breast or a small colon cancer would not have been noticed by a physician seventy-five years ago without the modern technology that we have today. However, visit the cancer ward at your local hospital. You will find patients there with advanced stages of cancer, and even a simple physical exam is all that is necessary to know that they have cancer. You can't miss a large ulcerating mass in a woman's breast, or an emaciated jaundiced patient with an enlarged, rock-hard irregular liver filled with cancer nodules. It does not take a rocket scientist to recognize the advanced stages of cancer."

Another interesting statistic was that well over 50 percent of cancer deaths in the early 1900s were gastrointestinal, and most of these were stomach cancers. For instance, Sir William Osler reported that of the first 8,464 admissions at Johns Hopkins, 150 were for stomach cancer![1] By comparison, I see stomach cancer today only once every couple of years, despite having a busy GI referral practice. Why was there so much stomach cancer a hundred years ago, yet it is uncommon today?

This is my theory. Recall that the stomach is like a gas tank for a car. Food sits there for up to ten or twelve hours before it completely empties out into your small intestine (which is why you should fast for twelve hours before surgery). Then recall that smoked meat was a staple a hundred years ago because there was no refrigeration, salt was relatively expensive and not always available, and smoking was the least expensive way to preserve meats. Also, fresh meat was often cooked over an open charcoal fire. In essence, then, smoked meats and charcoal-prepared food sat in people's stomachs for up to twelve hours after each meal. We also know that charcoal is high in carcinogens (cancer-causing substances), so this would explain why there was a lot of gastric cancer back then.

Presumably, this may also explain why until recently gastric cancer was the number one cause of cancer deaths in Southeast Asia.[2] Because people in the nineteenth century ate a high-fiber diet, I presume that once their food exited their stomach, it moved quickly through the rest of their intestinal tract. Any carcinogens or other toxins in the diet would likely be eliminated from their body before these substances could be appreciably absorbed. Also, any carcinogens and toxins in their diet would be avidly bound by the insoluble fiber so abundant in their food.

To me, the fiber program and healthy bowel habits are of such importance to general good health that such speculations about the possible prevention of cancer are simply a possible bonus to a diet rich in fiber. More scientific research will have to determine whether my observations hold any water. Dr. Denis Burkitt found solid epidemiological evidence that a healthy high-fiber diet and excellent bowel program will help prevent gallbladder disease, coronary artery disease, hiatal hernia and reflux, appendicitis, varicose veins, hemorrhoids, diverticulitis, and colon cancer. Why didn't Burkitt consider other types of cancer and Alzheimer's disease preventable with the fiber program? I can only guess. We do know that Alzheimer's disease began to become widely prevalent in the Western hemisphere in the 1970s, so its arrival was probably too late in his career to study (he died in 1993 at age eighty-two). Also, Burkitt built his reputation by describing what later became known as Burkitt's lymphoma. In 1964, this cancer was found to be caused by the Epstein-Barr virus. Since by the 1960s, science had demonstrated that viruses, certain toxins (e.g. radiation, arsenic, cobalt), and genes could cause cancer, I suspect that this may have affected his decision not to study other cancers, thinking that there was an adequate explanation for the majority of cancers in the Western hemisphere.

Although I agree with many of Burkitt's conclusions, this book is about what I have learned during my many years working as a gastroenterologist. In essence, Burkitt and I looked at the same questions, but from different viewpoints, so our findings would be expected to vary. Burkitt worked as a missionary surgeon to Africa in the middle part of the twentieth century for more than two decades, whereas I began practicing as a GI doctor in the United States in 1983, with brief annual visits to South America. What we saw as clinicians and what we read in the scientific literature were different, and this explains why our conclusions vary. But we emphatically agreed on the critical nature of a good fiber program for long-term good health.

Your Body's Unique Filtration Systems

Everybody who has an aquarium understands the importance of the filtration system for clear water and healthy fish. But although the filtration system is important, even more important is the need to replace the filters periodically. The human body is much more complicated than an aquarium but similar in many ways. The body has about a half dozen different filtration systems designed to keep your body in as good health as possible. Most everyone knows about the importance of the kidneys for filtering the blood, eliminating waste products and other harmful chemicals. Anyone who has lived with kidney failure and then received a kidney transplant can attest to the importance of the kidneys for general good health; even the most advanced dialysis machines cannot equal the work your kidneys do. Your blood is also constantly being filtered by your spleen and liver.

Another filtration system is the lymphatic system, which acts as a barrier to prevent serious infections and cancer from spreading. Each lymph node acts like a filter, trapping aberrant bacteria and cancer cells. Excess fluid in your legs is returned to your bloodstream when your lymphatic system is operating as it should, preventing your legs from swelling. A bad heart or prolonged standing or inactivity, especially combined with obesity, disrupts your lymphatic system in addition to the venous drainage system of your legs. The spleen works somewhat like a giant lymph node but filters your blood directly.

Your liver is a key player in operating the *enterohepatic circulation*, another very important filtration system. *Entero-* means "gut" and *hepatic* means "liver." Bile circulates continuously between your liver and your intestines. Your bile is first secreted by your liver and then stored and concentrated in your gallbladder. When you eat, your gallbladder contracts and empties your bile via the bile duct into your small intestine. There, your bile helps you digest and absorb your food, and then it returns by your portal vein to your liver to start the cycle all over again. Enterohepatic circulation is second only to your kidneys in importance. Although your lymphatic system and spleen also act as filtration systems, only your kidneys and your enterohepatic circulation allow the body to rid itself of any noxious substances. Because your enterohepatic circulation operates by an entirely different system than your kidneys, the types of chemicals and toxins that it removes are quite different from those removed by your kidneys.

There are other filtration and circulatory systems in the body, including the cerebral fluid (brain and spinal fluid) and even the aqueous system of your eye. So the human body has a number of filtration systems in place that are critical to good long-term health. Think of the Sea of Galilee and the Dead Sea in Israel. Both are large bodies of water that are interconnected by the Jordan River. The Sea of Galilee is brimming with life, but only eighty miles to the south and connected by the same river, the Dead Sea is just that, even though it is much larger. Why the difference? The Jordan River flows completely through the Sea of Galilee with constant inflow and outflow, whereas the Jordan River ends at the Dead Sea, which has no outlet other than by way of evaporation, sitting at 1,300 feet below sea level. Water continuously evaporates out of the Dead Sea, leaving behind salt and other minerals that are so concentrated that they are toxic to all but the hardiest life forms. Only brine shrimp and a few plants can survive in this harsh environment. In fact, the salt content of the Dead Sea is estimated to be nine times that of the Atlantic Ocean!

Thinking of your body in this way allows you to appreciate the importance of multiple effective filtration systems for good health, but even more important than filtration is the means by which waste and toxic products can be ejected out of the body. Your kidneys and enterohepatic circulation have an effect similar to the Jordan River flowing through the Sea of Galilee, allowing the inflow and outflow of water and other chemical substances, in essence completely replacing the water in your aquarium (your body) as well as the filters and even vacuuming out the bottom as well. Although your lymphatic system and spleen (and your other filtration systems) are important filters for your body's aquarium, they are not considered as essential for your survival. As an example, people who have their spleens removed generally live a healthy life. The reason is that the body has backup systems that can compensate for losing your spleen. Not so when your kidneys or liver stop working as they should.

Knowing that your kidneys and liver are essential in ridding the body of any toxic wastes, you won't be surprised that cancer is more common in people with chronic kidney disease and cirrhosis (end-stage liver disease, in which the liver is scarred and on the verge of failure). Cirrhosis is associated with an especially striking increase in cancer risk. Research has shown that all types of cirrhosis are associated with a high risk of liver cancer (hepatocellular carcinoma)—so high that physicians caring for patients with cirrhosis consider routine annual screening of their patients with ultrasounds and blood work in order to catch this devastating cancer at an early phase.

Conventional thinking has it that liver cancer can be attributed to liver injury, but one must wonder whether the failing enterohepatic circulation, which is so dependent on normal liver function, may play a contributory role. I am not aware of research indicating an increase in other types of cancer (that is, cancers outside the liver) in patients with cirrhosis, but I would expect to find such an increase. It would be an easy hypothesis to test.

Research has shown that both hepatitis B and C viruses (HBV and HCV) may live for years in the liver and other organ tissues without causing any apparent harm to the body. I am currently following a patient who has had two liver biopsies fifteen years apart without any evidence of liver damage caused by his HCV infection. His risk of developing liver cancer would be very low for this reason. Indeed, liver cancer is much less common if you do not have cirrhosis, even if you have had HBV or HCV for decades—the primary exception being if you were infected at birth with HBV. However, if HBV or HCV has caused cirrhosis, then you have a much higher risk of developing liver cancer. Indeed, liver cancer is one of the most rapidly increasing cancers in the United States. Moreover, fatty livers caused by the obesity epidemic in the United States are also causing a rapidly rising incidence of cirrhosis and liver cancer. In fact, annual screening for liver cancer is recommended for most individuals with cirrhosis, whether it is caused by a fatty liver, HBV or HCV, or other liver diseases such as hemachromatosis.

Looking at these statistics, I cannot help but ask myself, how does bile uncouple itself from toxic chemicals once it has moved them to the intestine? Pick up a can of Metamucil. What does the label say? "If you are taking a prescription medicine, take this product at least 2 hours before or after the prescribed medicine." Why does the Metamucil container say this? Because high-quality fiber like that in Metamucil binds everything in sight. I advise parents that their children should not get their fiber during their most nutritious meals, because absorption of vitamins and other nutrients would probably be impaired. This is probably partly why people in developing countries where there is a far greater proportion of quality fiber in the diet are so much shorter than folks in economically advanced nations: because essential nutrients and vitamins get swept out of their system before they can be absorbed.

So you should think of quality fiber such as bran and Metamucil as "scrubbing" your bile, thereby removing toxic wastes or chemicals and preventing them from being recycled back into the body as your bile is reabsorbed. Recall the difference between the Sea of Galilee and the Dead Sea. I read somewhere that the colon is capable of absorbing up to 2,000 calories daily. In fact, there was a case report of a fourteen-year-old girl who had had all but six inches of her small bowel surgically removed, but she managed because her colon was left intact, which allowed her to absorb the nutrients she needed to live.[3] If the colon can absorb healthy nutrients, it is reasonable to postulate that carcinogens and other toxins in undigested foodstuffs (the leftovers) can be absorbed as well. If you don't "scrub" those toxins from your bile, over time your body will inch from being the Sea of Galilee toward becoming like the Dead Sea. That's my theory, at any rate.

But there is a second hidden benefit here, and that is that good-quality fiber accelerates the exiting of your undigested food waste out of the body and makes your stools bulkier. Whatever chemicals and toxins move through your gut are therefore not as concentrated and are out of your body in a matter of hours rather than days or weeks, making them less likely to be absorbed by your gut. Similarly, there would be a decreased production of chemical carcinogens by bacterial flora in the gut as well. I tell my patients to think of bran and Metamucil as pre-emergent weed killers; good-quality fiber helps prevent the weeds (such as tumors and cancers) before they have a chance to take root in the body. In the 1980s, I performed several colonoscopies and removed more than eighty polyps in a middle-aged man. Five years later, he returned for a follow-up exam and I could not find a single polyp! It seems that he had been eating his bran cereal in the morning and having Metamucil at night ever since his first visit to my office.

This chapter suggests that two of the most frightening scourges of the late twentieth century—cancer and Alzheimer's disease—may be preventable or at least delayed in onset. Dr. Denis Burkitt would go further. Drawing on his own epidemiologic research, he was convinced that fiber was central to the prevention of coronary heart disease. If people took to the high-fiber diet, he felt that coronary heart disease might be eradicated. Yet the medical profession pays only lip service to the importance of high-quality fiber, in large part because the high-fiber diet has been so poorly understood. I hope to bring the spotlight back on fiber as a low-cost way to prevent high-cost medical problems. I think that doctors should not just check your blood pressure; they should also check on your bowel habits and ask whether you are on a quality fiber program. Remember, not just any fiber will do, and don't forget what the fiber is supposed to do in the bathroom.

But processed white flour does not itself cause cancer. I have no hesitation about eating processed flour products such as pasta and bread, as long as I have an adequate amount of high-quality fiber intake daily. Rather, I suspect that the fiber in whole-grain wheat products helps protect us from cancer.

The world is a dangerous place, full of harmful things that may hurt and even kill us. However, when people eat insufficient amounts of insoluble fiber, they are hampering one of the natural filtration processes from working as effectively as it should (the enterohepatic circulation).

Thoughts on Prevention of Alzheimer's Disease

Alzheimer's disease is a frightening illness; studies suggest that up to 10 percent of Americans over age sixty-five and 50 percent of Americans over age eighty-five have at least early Alzheimer's disease. Research has shown that a certain genetic heritage is responsible for most cases of Alzheimer's disease, and in fact today you can have yourself tested for the Alzheimer's gene. But not all individuals who have the genetic makeup develop Alzheimer's disease, nor does everyone who develops it have the genetic code. For these reasons, scientists believe that at least a second major factor must be involved in the development of this illness. Current thinking is that this second factor may be environmental.

In the 1990s, several reports surfaced describing a high incidence of Alzheimer's-like illnesses in dialysis patients being given aluminum-containing antacids. Prior to these reports, these antacids were widely prescribed for patients with kidney failure. These products have now been all but withdrawn from routine use in dialysis patients. But I was struck by how quickly these antacids seemed to cause this Alzheimer's-like illness. Periodically I see dialysis patients, and I have noted how often these patients are constipated.

I also realized that I had never seen any patients with Alzheimer's disease in Bolivia. Dr. Dardo Chávez and other physicians have confirmed to me that this disease is indeed rare, and absent in the Montero/Santa Cruz area where I work. With this in mind, one day at Cape Fear Valley Medical Center here in Fayetteville I approached an aging neurologist, Dr. Martin Chipman, who has practiced neurology since the 1950s, and told him, "I am willing to wager that Alzheimer's disease did not commonly exist in the United States fifty years ago as it does today." Dr. Chipman looked at me with interest and said, "You are correct. There are several theories as to why this is the case." He postulated that Alzheimer's disease may have been common fifty years ago, but the culture of our society at the time was to ignore the problem rather than to seek treatment.

Subsequently, a retired forensic pathologist (one who does autopsies) who practiced during the 1970s commented to me that he recalls receiving the body of a person with the Alzheimer's diagnosis in 1978. He had never heard of this disorder before and remembered having to get his medical textbooks out to read about the illness. Two retired internists, Dr. Weldon Jordan and Dr. Malcolm Fleishman, who also began practicing in the 1950s, both recall that Alzheimer's disease was virtually unheard of until the 1970s. Dr. Chipman also indicated that the prevalence of Alzheimer's disease has greatly increased in recent years, and he also stated that it is significantly more common today than only fifteen years ago.

Since that conversation with Dr. Chipman, I have been waiting for Alzheimer's disease to arrive in Bolivia. Sure enough, in 2005, while I was visiting a clinic in El Alto, a city on the Altiplano just outside La Paz, the physicians at a CSRA clinic there confirmed that Alzheimer's disease indeed was now in the La Paz and El Alto region of Bolivia. Dr. Esperanza Aid, a retired dentist, said, "There are no statistics in Bolivia. No one really knows what is going on here." However, Dr. Aid did confer with some of her medical colleagues, and their impression is that Alzheimer's disease arrived in the La Paz/El Alto area only at the beginning of the twenty-first century, or within the past ten years.

My physician contacts in the Santa Cruz/Montero area of Bolivia still maintain that Alzheimer's disease is not there. This is not surprising because Santa Cruz and Montero are considered nouveau riche areas of Bolivia, and for this reason I would anticipate Alzheimer's disease to arrive there later than it did in La Paz if indeed dietary fiber plays a role in the evolution of this illness. The population of Santa Cruz alone now exceeds one million. Further, in July 2005, when I met with gastroenterologists from the Montero/Santa Cruz area to discuss my fiber program and fiber hypotheses, I relayed my concern that I expect Alzheimer's disease to arrive there soon, probably within a decade. There are likely other possible reasons why Alzheimer's disease was so late to arrive in Bolivia, but if so, it is not common knowledge to my physician contacts there. Remember that until a few hundred years ago, people thought the world was flat and that the sun rotated around the earth. Association does not mean causality. But there are a few other pieces of circumstantial evidence to consider.

Indeed, over the years, several other scientific studies have also implicated aluminum as a possible second contributing factor. Aluminum has been found in the plaques that are part of the pathology of the brain of a person with Alzheimer's disease. Whether aluminum causes the illness or is just an innocent bystander is a question that has been debated for years. One objection to the aluminum hypothesis is that the nerve damage that occurs when aluminum is injected into the brains of animals is different from what is seen in Alzheimer's disease.[4] But trying to study Alzheimer's disease by studying the effects of aluminum injected directly into the brain is not comparable. Skin damaged by forty years of exposure to the sun looks different from simple sunburn, but the cause of both is the same—UV light exposure. A second argument against the aluminum hypothesis is that studies have shown that brain aluminum levels increase with aging in everyone.

My position is that if you have the right genetic makeup *and* high brain aluminum levels, you are more likely to develop the illness, whereas if you do not have the right genetic makeup *or* if you do not have high brain aluminum levels, then perhaps you will not develop Alzheimer's disease. It would be interesting to learn whether anyone has looked at brain aluminum levels from people who died seventy-five years ago, when Alzheimer's disease was rare. (Some human brains from that era are still being kept in a few labs across the country.)

Not surprisingly, I also found that the scientific literature confirmed my suspicions that Alzheimer's disease is much less prevalent in developing nations. But then again, developing nations also have a great many fewer neurologists. However, Dr. H. C. Hendrie and colleagues reported that black people of African descent living in the United States were more than twice as likely to develop Alzheimer's disease as their ethnic and genetic counterparts in Nigeria, based on his own research studies,[5] once again lending credence to the idea that environmental factors must be contributing to the development of this illness in addition to genetic makeup. I believe that as with the development of cancer in Western societies, if you are genetically disposed to Alzheimer's disease, when the level of a certain toxic compound in the human body is reached, you will start to see the beginnings of the disease's symptoms. This chemical may well be aluminum, but other metals or minerals may be involved.

If aluminum is this second environmental cofactor, then it would stand to reason that anything that may affect aluminum's absorption by the gut would affect the prevalence of this illness. This is where my fiber hypothesis kicks in. If there is slow gut transit, with high concentrations of aluminum (or any other metal or mineral) in the diet, Alzheimer's disease may develop. By the same logic in which I discussed the prevention of cancer, these minerals will be absorbed less if the diet is loaded with high-quality fiber. We already know that a high-fiber diet undermines the body's ability to absorb nutrients, so why should it not also work to prevent the absorption of bad minerals?

Therefore, I expect that Mormons not only develop less cancer than other Americans, but also have less Alzheimer's disease. I have not been able to find information supporting or contradicting this expectation. This is especially curious because Mormons are reported to live longer than the average U.S. citizen and because we know that the prevalence of Alzheimer's disease rapidly increases as one ages. However, while researching causes of death among the Amish, who grind their own wheat, I found that not only do the Amish have a much lower prevalence of cancer, but they also have a much lower incidence of Alzheimer's disease.

An apparent problem with the fiber hypothesis is that the arrival of Alzheimer's disease occurred some fifty years after the arrival of cancer in the United States. If fiber is the key to unlocking the clues to this illness, then I would expect to see Alzheimer's disease becoming prevalent back during the middle part of the twentieth century, rather than in the 1970s. I subsequently found that aluminum foil was first introduced in 1913 for wrapping candy and gum.

But I was more struck with the timing of the arrival of aluminum cans in 1956 in the United States. Recall that many carbonated sodas have a very low pH. It would stand to reason that aluminum may ever so slowly be leached out of aluminum cans, especially if the beverages were not consumed soon after production. This could easily be proved or disproved by a simple test for aluminum content in a cola stored in a can for six months or so versus one fresh out of the factory. I myself have periodically noticed a distinctly metallic taste in beverages stored in aluminum cans. Because the factories that manufacture aluminum cans are expensive to build, and because of shipping costs, I suspect that the arrival of Alzheimer's disease in the La Paz area of Bolivia may be correlated with the antecedent arrival of aluminum-containing beverages only two or three decades earlier.

I could not find anything about aluminum pots, but they almost certainly arrived much earlier than the aluminum can because the manufacturing process would likely not be as sophisticated. Also, food prepared in an aluminum pot would likely be stored at most only a few days, whereas beverages prepared for shipping in aluminum cans would likely sit months before consumption. Some people may argue that food cooked in aluminum pots may absorb aluminum more readily than the beverages in a soda can. My thought here is that aluminum ions would more easily be leached out by the much higher acidity of beverages, and also that the diffusion process would occur more readily in a liquid beverage than in regular food stored in an aluminum pot. A better way to explain this would be to throw a tablespoon of salt on a meat loaf. You can shake the meat loaf, but the only way to really mix the salt would be to mash up the meat loaf in order for the salt to be evenly distributed. Not so for a bottle of soda. Throw in a tablespoon of salt, shake the bottle a couple of times, and bingo! The salt is evenly distributed throughout. In essence, the diffusion process would occur much more readily in a liquid than in semi-solid or solid food. So although aluminum pots may be a second potential way to be exposed to dietary aluminum, I suspect that aluminum beverage cans would be the primary source of exposure. A chemist would best be able to address this question, however. Another interesting observation is that people who subsist on well water with high aluminum levels have a high incidence of developing an Alzheimer's-like illness.

To the scientific community, the conclusions drawn in this chapter are mere speculation. And I must admit that the line of thought woven herein is based on a few odd observations that, when combined with a smattering of scientific facts, lead to startling conclusions. However, if one considers that high-quality fiber diets are a potential low-cost solution for preventing or delaying the onset of the more costly and common catastrophic illnesses among the middle-aged and elderly, everyone should take pause. Although this chapter suggests that two of the most frightening scourges of the late twentieth century may indeed be preventable, noteworthy is the fact that even the late Dr. Denis Burkitt himself was convinced that high-fiber diets were central to the prevention of numerous illnesses common to Western society, based on his own careful epidemiological studies throughout the world only three decades ago.

KEY POINTS TO REMEMBER

- Elie Metchnikoff first proposed autointoxication as the cause of numerous degenerative illnesses more than a century ago.

- Cancer first became widely prevalent in the Montero/ Santa Cruz area of Bolivia in 1995 and became well entrenched in the United States by 1950. Both events occurred roughly thirty years after the widespread arrival of processed flour.

- Like an aquarium, your body uses filtration systems to remove toxic waste materials. Dietary fiber scrubs your bile as it circulates in your body, which is second in importance only to your kidneys in ejecting toxins outside your body.

- An Alzheimer's-like illness rapidly developed in kidney dialysis patients taking aluminum-containing antacids.

- Alzheimer's disease first became widely recognized in the United States in the 1970s and is just now beginning to arrive in the old wealth areas of Bolivia.

- Dietary aluminum *and* a low-fiber diet may act as cofactors with your genetic background, causing Alzheimer's disease.

- The theory that most cancers and Alzheimer's disease are preventable illnesses (or can be significantly delayed in onset) with a high-quality fiber program should be carefully studied. Prevention is vastly less expensive than treating a problem once it arises.

Notes

1. Osler W. *The Principles and Practice of Medicine.* 4th ed. New York, NY: Appleton & Company; 1902.

2. Gastric cancer was the number one cause of cancer death worldwide until the 1980s, only overtaken in the 1980s by lung cancer, mostly because there was so much gastric cancer in developing nations, including Southeast Asia.

3. Anderson CM. Long-term survival with six inches of small intestine. *Br Med J.* 1965;1(5432):406-4, 419–422.

4. Keizner LJ. Diagnosis and treatment of Alzheimer's disease *Adv Intern Med.* 1984;29:447–470.

5. Hendrie HC, Hall KS, Ogunniyi A, Gao S. Alzheimer disease: genes and environment; The value of international studies. *Can J Psychiatry.* 2004;49(2):92–99.

Afterword

Having spent more than twenty-five years in private practice in Fayetteville, North Carolina, and being involved in international health care for almost as many years, I have become convinced of the absolute importance of ownership of ideas by individuals and their communities. It doesn't matter how rational a proposed health care intervention is; if the person and the community don't take ownership, then the idea is lost in the flood of information that we receive every day.

A case study that expounds on this concept involving ownership of ideas and its relevancy to this book is Curamericas Global, Inc., a small nonprofit international health care organization with projects in Bolivia, Guatemala, and more recently in Haiti and Liberia. To date, all of the projects that we have initiated since Curamericas' founding more than a quarter century ago are still operational and self-sustaining despite their location in impoverished areas and despite our own limited financial support. Curamericas is now taking note, and we believe that community ownership of our projects is why we have been successful, what we call building social capital. How did this happen and how does this relate to my book, *Cure Constipation Now*? A bit of Curamericas Global history will explain.

Fifty years ago, as a young physician, the late John Wyon, professor emeritus at the Harvard School of Public Health, learned that neonatal tetanus was a preventable but highly fatal illness in impoverished nations. On his first visit to India, when Dr. Wyon asked about neonatal tetanus, he was told that the illness was rare. A few months later, when he visited the surrounding villages, he found that babies were dying by the thousands of this illness. He concluded that if you don't visit the poor in their homes, you will not know what the real public health challenges are. And if you don't measure the impact of your interventions, you will have no idea of how effective your treatments are. Hence he developed the concept of the census-based, impact-oriented (CBIO) approach. A nonprofit that uses the CBIO methodology will regularly go to every home in the community, keeping computer records to track the health care of the families and measuring the impact of the health care provided.

But just as important, because we have made this information available to the communities we serve, they have taken ownership of our projects. With the CBIO approach, they now have vision. They can see where they were two or three years ago, where they are today, and where they hope to be in the near future using the statistical information that the CBIO approach provides. This means that our communities and project leaders will make every effort to marshal their own resources to keep our projects going if and when our funding dries up—resources that Curamericas Global could never tap otherwise.

As an example, after twenty-five years in Bolivia our projects are now finally close to becoming self-sustaining. Sustainability took only five years in Guatemala. There, Dr. Mario Valdez, our project director, quickly grasped the significance of the CBIO approach, and he has been actively marketing our findings to the communities we serve. Rates of maternal and infant deaths, use of oral rehydration formulas for diarrhea, and vaccination rates for the community are even posted at the city hall. We believe that this approach may transform international health care.

How does this relate to this book? Everybody knows that high-fiber diets are important to general good health, though the reason for this is poorly understood by almost everyone. This is similar to Curamericas using CBIO methodology for almost twenty-five years without recognizing its full potential. I hope now that you have come to understand the critical relationship among good health, a good fiber program, and healthy bowel habits, you will take ownership of my message in much the same way as the people did in our communities in Bolivia and Guatemala. Solid scientific evidence shows that a high-quality fiber diet prevents or reduces the incidence of reflux, gallbladder disease, appendicitis, hemorrhoids, diverticulitis, varicose veins, and coronary heart disease, not to mention its other benefits to GI health. I also firmly believe that the onset of most cancers and Alzheimer's disease can be either prevented or significantly delayed with a high-quality fiber program.

Sometime during my medical training I learned that half of all health care expenditures are directly related to poor lifestyle choices: obesity, smoking, and drinking alcohol to excess. Theoretically, at least, health care costs could be reduced by half if people choose to pursue healthier lifestyles. Now, because a good fiber program can prevent many if not most of the preceding illnesses, and perhaps also cancer and Alzheimer's disease, might it also be possible that two-thirds or even three-fourths of our health care costs could be preventable if a good fiber program were added to this list of healthy lifestyle choices? Many Americans have chosen the first three—staying trim and fit, not smoking, and using alcohol in moderation—but are completely unaware of the fourth, a good fiber program, and its benefits to health. Do you want to keep this a secret any longer?

Years ago, I was giving my fiber spiel to a young country girl in Bolivia with abdominal gas issues. At the conclusion of the conversation, she excitedly told me that as soon as she got home to her village she was going to tell her mother, her sister, her aunt, and her grandmother what I had just told her. In essence, I had a new convert to my fiber program. I half-jokingly tell my patients that I am raising up an army of folks taking bran and Metamucil. I say, "We are going to take over the world." I also tell them that I am trying to change the world's thinking about bathroom habits, and I cannot do it by myself. I need help.

But we also need to understand that although almost 80 million U.S. citizens have chronic GI problems, another 150 million U.S. citizens don't even realize they have a lurking problem. The 80 million folks with the chronic GI issues are like my back, which likes to complain a lot and thereby keeps me out of trouble by making me do yoga and Pilates daily. But the other 150 million U.S. citizens' GI tracts are like my neck, which never likes to complain and never lets me know that danger is nearby. Then boom! It happens. I had to have that urgent neck surgery. For you it may be a heart attack, a gallbladder attack, or chest pain that sends you to the emergency room but is found to be caused by reflux, caused partly because you aren't making all those necessary bathroom stops. Recall that just because your GI tract is not talking to you, this does not mean all is well in the basement. People who are not on a good-quality fiber program often never realize that major damage is being done to the foundations of their house of health, unless of course someone sticks their nose down there and notices that musty odor.

We need to sound the alarm! Everybody knows what hypertension can do to your health if left untreated. So everybody tries to make sure their blood pressure is under control. But it is not true with constipation and that less-than-sweet odor in your bathroom. By not alerting your family, friends, and neighbors as to the broad significance and implications of this problem, you have let your fears of impropriety and social awkwardness overwhelm what is the right thing to do to help those you care about. So leave your Metamucil or Benefiber can out on your kitchen countertop and use it as an icebreaker.

Tell them about this crazy doctor in Fayetteville, North Carolina, who thinks everybody should poop like a cow. You would not walk around with a garbage bag slung over your shoulder all day long, so why does everybody smile contentedly with a bag of the stuff just rotting away inside their GI tracts? Everybody knows that when they have better bathroom results, they feel better. It's not complicated. Then give your own modified version of my "fiber talk." You need to be on a mission like that young Bolivian woman. Talk to everybody who will listen. We have got to get this bathroom talk out of the bathroom NOW! and get this message out to people everywhere. Their health and quite possibly their lives will depend on it!

Index

Page numbers in **bold** indicate tables.